Secrets of a Healer - Magic of Advanced Aromatherapy

SECRETS OF A HEALER

VOL. IX
MAGIC OF ADVANCED AROMATHERAPY

Dr. Constance Santego

Maximillian Enterprises
Kelowna, BC

Ordering Information: Quantity sales. Special discounts are available on quantity purchases by corporations, associations, and others. For details, contact the "Special Sales Department" at the address above.

Copy Editor & Interior Design: Constance Santego
Book Layout: ©2017 BookDesignTemplates.com
Cover Design: Jennifer Louie
Second Edition Copyright 2020
Trade Paperback ISBN: 978-1-7772220-4-8
eBook ISBN 978-1-7772220-5-5
Published by Maximillian Enterprises
Kelowna, BC Canada
www.constancesantego.ca
Created and published In Canada. Printed and bound in the United States of America

Dedication

To all the Aromatherapy healers!

God gave us the ability to learn what we need to know on how to heal the body naturally!

−Dr. Constance Santego

ALSO BY DR. CONSTANCE SANTEGO

FICTION
The Nine Spiritual Gifts Series:

Journey of a Soul – (Vol. 1 Michael)
Language of a Soul – (Vol. 2 Gabriel)
Prophecy of a Soul – (Vol. 3 Bath Kol)
Healing of a Soul – (Vol. 4 Raphael)

NON-FICTION
The Intuitive Life, The Gift of Prophecy, Third Edition

Fairy Tales, Dreams and Reality... Where Are You On Your Path?
Second Edition
Your Persona... The Mask You Wear
Angelic Lifestyle, A Vibrant Lifestyle
Angelic Lifestyle 42-Day Energy Cleanse
Archangel Michael's Soul Retrieval Guide

SECRETS OF A HEALER, SERIES:

Magic of Aromatherapy (Vol. I)
Magic of Reflexology (Vol. II)
Magic of The Gifts (Vol. III)
Magic of Muscle Testing (Vol. IV)
Magic of Iridology (Vol. V)
Magic of Massage (Vol. VI)
Magic of Hypnotherapy (Vol. VII)
Magic of Reiki (Vol. VIII)
Magic of Advanced Aromatherapy (Vol. IX)
Magic of Esthetics (Vol. X)

FOR CHILDREN

I am big tonight. I don't need the light!

Contents

Note to Reader.. xiii

Learning Outcome.. xv

Advanced Aromatherapy..1

    Neuropathic Pain & Cause 4

Body Systems.. 12

    Cardiovascular System 13

    Digestive System 15

    Endocrine System 17

    Immune System...21

    Integumentary System/Skin......................................23

    Lymphatic System..38

    Muscular System..41

    Neurological System 44

    Reproductive System..47

    Respiratory System 50

    Skeletal System..52

    Urinary System..53

    TCRS ESO For Each System Of The Body...............55

How Essential Oils are Tested for Quality 59

    Time of Harvest!!!..70

Chemical Components of an Essential Oil 78

    Chemical Structure 78

    Single Covalent Bond...93

    Double Covalent Bond 94

Molecular Compounds..................................... 95

Biochemistry 96

    Organic Chemistry 96

    Written Formula of a Bond........................ 101

Functional Groups/ Chemical Families 112

    List of Essential Oils in each Family..... 114

    Hydrocarbons 115

    Monoterpenes 116

    Sesquiterpenes 120

    Diterpenes 124

    Alcohols 125

    Monoterpenols.. 125

    Sesquiterpenols... 129

    Diterpenols 131

    Phenols... 132

    Aldehydes... 135

    Ketones 139

    Acids.. 143

    Esters... 145

    Ethers 147

    Oxides.. 149

    Lactones... 152

    Coumarins.. 154

    Furocoumarins 155

Chemical Overview... 156

Advanced Aromatherapy Procedure.................... 157

Miscellaneous... 161

    Grid System... 161

    About Rosemary Caddy 164

    Aromatherapy and Cancer............................ 166

Bonus: Hydrotherapy for Pain 168

    Rules of Hydrotherapy................................. 170

Glossary 185

BIBLIOGRAPHY 210

MESSAGE FROM THE AUTHOR......................... 215

Note to Reader

Aromatherapy is not to replace modern medicine; Your Doctor still plays an essential role in your health care. For example, if I break my leg, I will need a Doctor and all the nurses and staff that work in the Hospitals to help me.

I believe Eastern Medicine believes that we play a major role in taking care of our health, not leaving it up to the doctors to fix us after the fact. Eastern Medicine is about balancing the body, mind, and soul, reducing our stress level, creating a vital energy force, and watching what we put into our body and mind.

Aromatherapy is a tool, a healing gift from nature, a technique that permits the well-being of our Body, Mind & Soul.

Shift happens...Create magic!

Learning Outcome

Advanced Aromatherapy uses the highest percentage of the appropriate chemical constituents of essential oil listed under the TCRS properties.

When you have completed this book and studied the concepts and techniques, you will.

- ➢ Know the basics of chemical constituents.
- ➢ How to find the highest percentage of the appropriate chemical constituents of an essential oil listed under the TCRS properties.
- ➢ Have an opportunity to create the BEST possible blend for yourself and your family's physical, mental, emotional, and spiritual body.

Advanced Aromatherapy

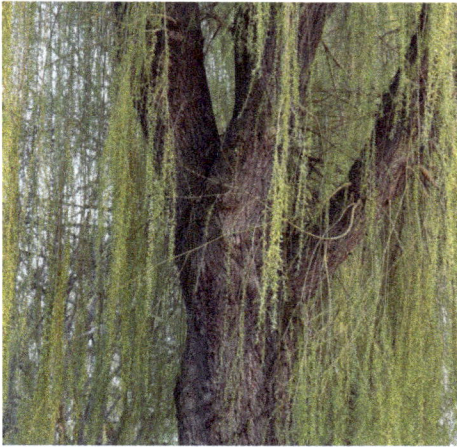

Did you know that Aspirin is made by taking the required chemical constituents for relieving pain from the bark of a willow tree?

But what is the specific constituent that relieves pain?

In the original Secrets of a Healer – Magic of Aromatherapy book, you learned how to choose essential oils using the Therapeutic Cross-Referencing information (acute, chronic, and synergistic recipes).

Many essential oils are listed under the top, middle, and base columns of the condition. Which one do you choose?

The one that helps all the conditions is preferred.
But how do you know it is the best essential oil to use?

In this Advance Aromatherapy book, you will learn how to choose the essential oil by the percentage of chemical constituents. The higher the percentage of the constituent (specific chemicals) listed in the functional group, the greater the healing effects.

Example:
We will continue with the essential oils best to relieve pain. If you have a person in pain, you want to alleviate their symptoms as quickly as possible.

When you go to the condition listed in the Therapeutic Cross-Referencing information and look under pain, you will find many top, middle, and base notes. And if the client did not have any contraindications, you could choose any of them.

BUT if you looked up the essential oils under their chemical constituents and noticed which ones have the highest percent of *acids, esters, aliphatic aldehydes,* and *ketones,* etc., you would have seen some constituents have a much higher **anti-inflammatory, anti-spasmodic, calming, and analgesic** property percentage than others. Meaning you would know and pick the essential oil(s) with a higher percentage of the chemical(s) needed in healing or helping the person's pain.

BUT, what type of pain is it? Pain is a symptom of many chronic or acute issues.

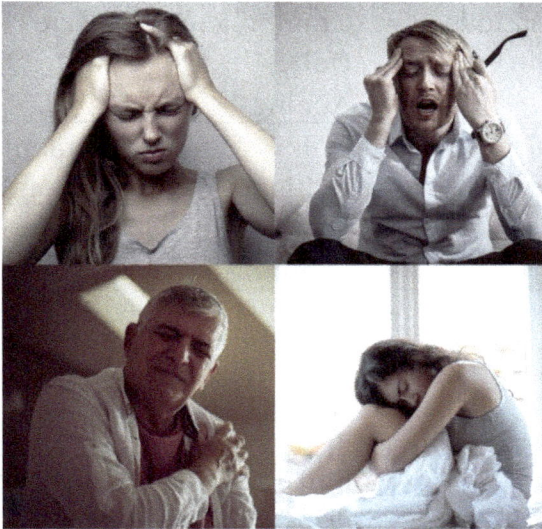

- Referred pain – may come from cutaneous (superficial tissue), somatic (including the skin, muscles, skeleton, joints, and connective tissues), visceral (organ), functional (when a patient presents with pain of no obvious organic origin - e.g., fibromyalgia), or psychological (emotional in origin, but experienced as organic).

Neuropathic Pain & Cause

Type	Symptom	Cause
Deep Somatic	• Cramping • Dull • Aching	Muscle
	• Dull • Aching	Ligament or Joint cap
Radicular	• Sharp • Shooting	Nerve root
	• Sharp • Bright • Lightening like	Nerve
	• Burning • Pressure like • Stinging • Aching	Sympathetic nerve
	• Deep • Nagging • Dull	Bone
	• Sharp • Sever • Intolerable	Fracture
Radicular	• Throbbing • Diffuse	Vasculature

Visceral	• Strong • Abnormal • GI contractions	Visceral (organ)
Stress	• Aches & pain • Anxiety • Change of appetite • Chronic fatigue • Difficulty sleeping • Irritability & impatience • Loss of interest & loss of enjoyment in life • Muscle tension (headaches) • Sweaty hands • Trembling • Withdrawal	

PAIN AND ITS RELATION TO THE SEVERITY OF REPETITIVE STRESS ACTIVITY

- Level 1 – Pain (Px) after a specific activity
- Level 2 – Px at the start of an action, resolving with the warm-up
- Level 3 – Px during and after a specific action that does not affect performance
- Level 4 – Px during and after a specific act that does affect performance
- Level 5 – Px with an activity of daily living (ADLs)
- Level 6 – Constant dull aching pain at rest that does not disturb sleep
- Level 7 – Dull aching pain that does disturb sleep

Do you know what the specific chemical constituent that relieves pain is? The active ingredient in the medicine made from willow bark is called salicin.

Salicin is an alcoholic β-glucoside
(2R,3S,4S,5R,6S)-2-(Hydroxymethyl)-6-[2-(hydroxymethyl) phenoxy] oxane-3, 4,5-triol

WHAT YOU LEARNED TO USE IN THE THERAPEUTIC CROSS-REFERENCING (TCRS) ESSENTIAL OIL CHOICES (BOOK 1 - MAGIC OF AROMATHERAPY)

Condition	Top Note	Middle Note	Base Note
Edema	Clary Sage	Fennel	Angelica
	Grapefruit	Geranium	
	Thyme	Cypress	
		Juniper	
		Rosemary	
		Lavender	
		Chamomile	

Condition	Top Note	Middle Note	Base Note
Aches and Pains	Basil	Black Pepper	Benzoin
	Cajuput	Camphor	Clove
	Caraway	Chamomile	Immortelle
	Coriander	Geranium	Nutmeg
	Eucalyptus	Juniper	
	Sage	Marjoram	
		Melissa	
		Peppermint	
		Rosemary	

Condition	Top Note	Middle Note	Base Note
Headaches	Eucalyptus	Chamomile	Immortelle
	Grapefruit	(R)	Linden
	Lemon	Lavender	Blossom
		Marjoram	Rose
		Melissa	
		Peppermint	
		Rosemary	
		Rosewood	

Recipes:

    Acute TMM

    Chronic MMB

    Synergistic TMB

If the person has no contraindications to these oils, you could use any of them, BUT, which oils have the most healing power for each condition?

BEST ESSENTIAL OILS FOR PAIN CAUSED BY:

Edema/Inflammation (Acute or Chronic)
    Property needed is **Anti-inflammatory**
    Constituent is **Monoterpenes / Sesquiterpene**

- Cedarwood 21-36%
- Hyssop 12%
- Juniper 60-80%
- Rosemary 15-37%
- Yarrow 5 -33.2%

Muscle Aches and Pain (Acute or Chronic)
    Property needed is **Relaxant, Anti-spasmodic**
    Constituent is **Monoterpenes, Esters, Sesquiterpene, Phenols, and Phenolic Ethers**

- Black Pepper 30-60%
- Ginger 11-51%
- Marjoram 20-50%
- Peppermint 16-36%

    Property needed is Analgesic
    Constituent is **Phenols and Phenolic Ethers**

- Aniseed 90-93%
- Black Pepper 30-60%
- Clove Bud 60-90%
- Fennel 50-90%
- Tarragon 60-75%

Headaches (Acute or Chronic)

Tension

Property needed is Analgesic

Constituent is **Phenols and Phenolic Ethers**

- Aniseed 90-93%
- Black Pepper 30-60%
- Clove Bud 60-90%
- Fennel 50-90%
- Tarragon 60-75%

Migraine

Property needed is Analgesic

Constituent is **Alcohols**

- Basil 40-55%
- Coriander 60-80%
- Geranium 55-65%
- Hyssop 47%
- Lavandin 23-48%
- Lemongrass 70-85%
- Marjoram 20-50%
- Neroli 30-40%
- Peppermint 16-36%
- Rose 22-60%
- Rosewood 82-95%
- Sandalwood 46-60%

NOW CHOOSE AN ESSENTIAL OIL based on the TCRS, BEST, if you understand the chemical constituent that makes up each essential oil.

Do not worry. The Advanced Aromatherapy procedure is easier than you think!

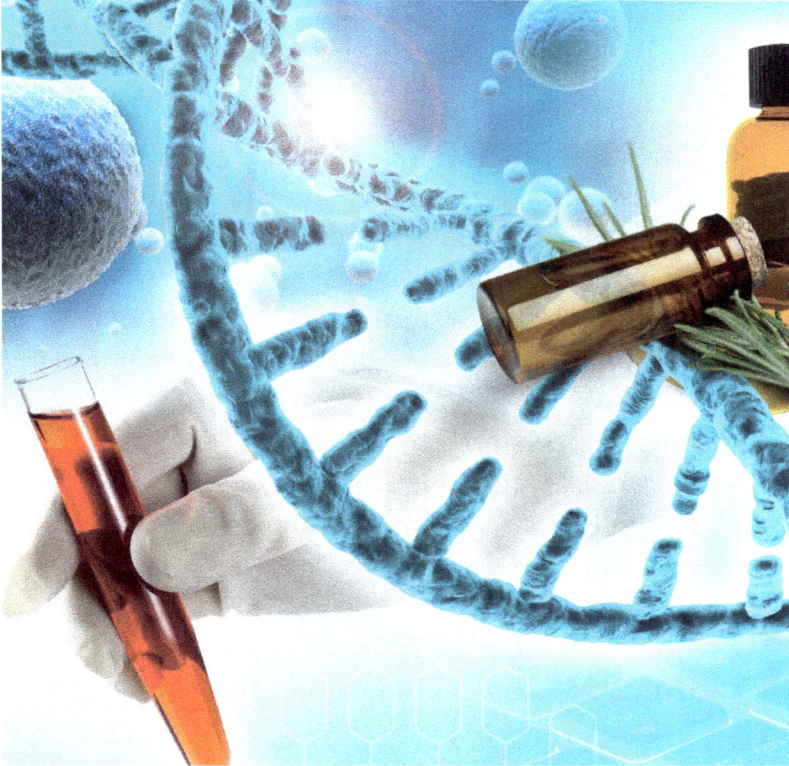

But first, you need to learn a few important facts.

Body Systems

- Cardiovascular System - blood
- Digestive System – nutrients and elimination
- Endocrine System – glands & hormones
- Immune System - disease
- Integumentary System/Skin - protection
- Lymphatic System – cellular garbage disposal & disease
- Muscular System - muscles
- Nervous System – Brain & messages
- Reproductive System – produces babies & hormones
- Respiratory System – breathing
- Skeletal System - bones
- Urinary System – elimination & water filtration

Cardiovascular System

Introduction

This system, also known as the circulatory system, consists of the heart, blood vessels, and blood. The center of the circulatory system is the heart, a muscular organ that rhythmically contracts, forcing the blood through a network of vessels.

Functions

The three functions of the system are to

- transport oxygen and nutrients to the cells
- remove metabolic wastes from the cells and tissues
- carry hormones from one part of the body to the other

Circulation

Circulation is the movement of blood from the heart to the lungs and back and to the rest of the body and back. Circulation is divided into two principal circuits, the **Systemic** or **General**

Circulation and the **Pulmonary Circulation.**
1. **Systemic** or **General** – the circulation from the ventricle to the rest of the body except the heart. The systemic circuit has two sub-circulatory branches. They are:

   a. **Hepatic Portal** – Normally, veins carry blood to the heart. However, the human body has a few veins that carry blood to the second set of exchange vessels. These veins are known as portal veins. The Hepatic Portal Vein or circulation carries blood from the digestive system to the liver. It starts on the intestine wall. Here tiny capillaries absorb nutrients. The blood flows to the hepatic portal vein, which gathers blood from the colon and the spleen. Next, the hepatic portal vein carries the blood to the liver. In the liver, liver cells remove nutrients whose concentrations are above homeostatic levels. The blood then joins the systemic circulation and is returned to the heart.

   b. **Cardiac or Coronary** -the circulation of blood to the heart muscle.

2. **Pulmonary** -blood circulation from the right ventricle to the lungs and back to the left atrium.

Digestive System

Introduction

The digestive system is one which people complain of the most. It is mistreated by the average person who insults it with poor quality food and water and inputs various toxic substances daily.

Functions

The function of the digestive system is:

- **To process food.** This function supplies nutrients to fuel the body's organs and systems.
- **To eliminate wastes from the body.**

General

This system is made up of mucous membranes like the type located in the respiratory and genito-urinary systems. The digestive system is a disassembly line that extracts vital parts from whole nutritional materials. It takes whole food products and breaks them down into chemical components. Digestive juices break down food into small, easily absorbed nutrients. In addition, they generate the energy required to maintain a healthy body.

The food content must be balanced and nutritious for a healthy and efficient working body to be maintained.

To a greater or lesser degree, we are responsible for our basic health. The old adage "we are what we eat" is often true. Because of this, we need to understand how it can go wrong.

The body requires raw material, heat, and energy to grow and repair itself. These raw materials are supplied in the form of food that comes in various packages that we ingest and convert to compounds, generating and sustaining life.

Endocrine System

Introduction

Endocrine means 'ductless.' This means the glands pass their secretions or hormones directly into the bloodstream, not through ducts like the gallbladder. The endocrine glands are distributed throughout the body and impact every function.

Function

The function of the overall system is to:

1. Regulate and integrate the body's metabolic activities.

2. Maintain homeostasis (balance). This is an organism or cell's ability or tendency to maintain internal equilibrium by adjusting its physiological processes.

System Parts

The endocrine system is made up of nine separate glands. They are the following:

1. hypothalamus
2. pituitary
3. pineal
4. thyroid
5. parathyroid
6. thymus
7. suprarenal or adrenals
8. part of the pancreas
9. parts of the ovaries and testes
10. placenta (when pregnant)

These glands work through the blood circulatory system and in conjunction with the nervous system. Each gland is separate in location. However, their functions are closely related to each other. The health of the body and, in many cases, the survival of the body is dependent upon the correct balanced output from the various glands.

Hormones

A hormone may be defined as:

- a substance that regulates bodily processes such as growth, metabolism, reproduction, and the functioning of various organs.

Hormones are secreted directly into the bloodstream by ductless or endocrine glands. The various glands maintain equilibrium among the hormones, producing their effects in very minute concentrations. They may pass through tissues unnoticed until they reach their target tissue. Only certain tissues will react to specific hormones.

When a hormone combines directly with the receptor, reactions occur. Because the hormone turns on a system or response called the first messenger. Some hormones are large molecules, and when they reach a target site, their presence activates enzymes that carry the message that turns on a response or system. These enzymes are called the second messenger.

Some hormones are steroids. These thyroid hormones are small molecules that can pass into the target cell. These can interact with DNA that activates certain genes and leads to the production of proteins. The proteins lead to changes in cells.

Hormones that stimulate other endocrine glands are called topical hormones.

Immune System

Introduction

The body's system is primarily responsible for destroying disease-causing agents in the immune system. This system is, perhaps, the most widespread system in our body. It functions everywhere.

Function

The immune system's function is:

- To defend the body against attack from infectious organisms and other harmful invaders (aka pathogens).
- Defense Systems

The immune system has three lines of defense. They are:
- physical and chemical barriers to infection (e.g., skin, mucous membranes),
- inflammatory response,
- immune response

Antigen

Any foreign substance that causes a reaction by the body's immune system is called an antigen.

Components and Specialized Cells

The system is not a neatly organized series of tubes and cells, such as the circulatory system. This system comprises a host of different cells and involves other systems. The other systems involved include:

- Lymphatic,
- Integument or skin,
- Endocrine.

The Threat

Four types of organisms can cause infection. They are:

- Viruses,
- Bacteria,
- Fungi,
- Parasites.

Integumentary System/Skin

Introduction

The skin is the largest organ in or on the body, and it has an especially important role to play in the absorbency of essential oils. The skin protects us and warns us of conditions interior and exterior of our bodies that may indicate a threat or condition we should be aware of.

The special senses are also an amazing aspect of our being, and although we may not be able to do a lot to help them with essential oils, we should be aware and actively working to maintain their health.

Skin or Integument

The skin is the largest organ or the body. Healthy skin is slightly moist, soft, and flexible and possesses a slight acid mantle. Its texture should be smooth and fine-grained. The color depends upon the blood supply and melanin content.

It is a protective organ covering the surface of the body. Without a break, it joins with the mucous membranes of the alimentary and other canals. The skin forms a protective barrier against the harmful effects of physical, chemical, and bacterial agents. It contains the end organs for the sense of touch. It maintains body temperature through the activity of its sweat glands and blood vessels.

The skin is an important organ. It has four primary functions:

1. Serves as a protective cover against invading pathogens
2. Regulates body temperatures via perspiration and shivering
3. Provides a waterproof covering for the body
4. Receives information about the outside world. It is the most distal part of the peripheral nervous system.

Diagram of the Skin

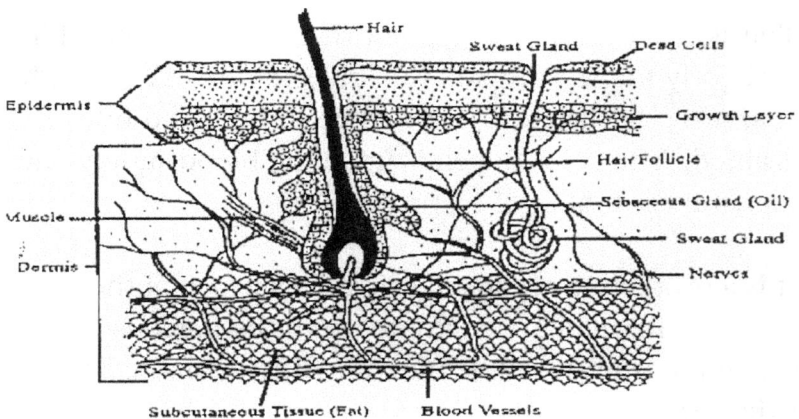

General

Skin is a large, elastic organ. The average human adult body is covered with about eighteen square feet of skin. It varies in thickness, being very thin over the eyelids and very thick on the soles of the feet. It weighs about seven pounds and provides excellent protection against germs, as very few can penetrate unbroken skin. The skin, except for a few areas such as the palms, soles, and ears, is loosely attached to the underlying tissues.

The color of the skin varies with the amount of pigmentation. The color varies during a disease because of the difference in pigment. In certain places, the outer layers of the skin are modified to produce hair and nails. The skin varies in thickness from 0.5 mm (0.02 in) on the eyelids to 4mm (0.17 in) or more on the palms and soles.

As an indication of the complexity of the skin, it has been estimated that one square centimeter of skin contains approximately:

- 65 hairs
- 95 - 100 sebaceous glands
- 78 yards of nerves
- 19 yards of blood vessels

- 650 sweat glands
- 9,500,000 cells
- 1,300 nerve endings to record pain
- 19,500 sensory cells at the end of nerve fibers
- 78 sensory apparatuses for heat
- 13 sensory apparatuses for cold
- 160 - 165 pressure apparatuses for the perception of tactile stimuli

The skin has two principal divisions; however, it consists of three distinct layers:

1. The **epidermis** is the outer layer of the skin, which contains nerve endings but no blood vessels. The tissue fluid derived from the dermis nourishes it. On average, it is about as thick as a page of a book. The epidermis consists of stratified epithelial tissue. The outermost cells wear and die and are constantly shed from the surface. It is like tree bark, with the cells growing from below it. New epidermal cells are constantly produced in the deepest sub-layer of the epidermis. The new cells mature and are pushed to the surface by new cells underneath. The cells at the surface are mostly filled with **keratin**. Keratin is a tough waterproof protein that makes the skin surface very water-resistant.

Epidermis - 5 layers

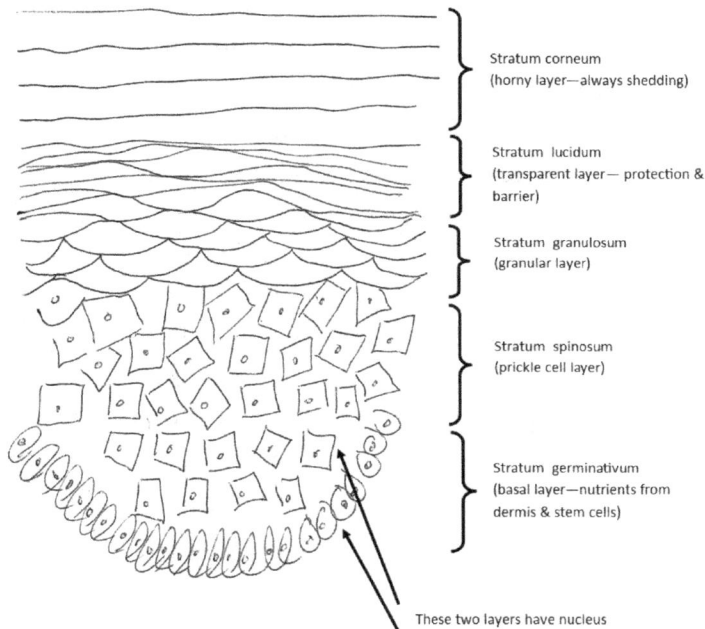

Stratum corneum
(horny layer—always shedding)

Stratum lucidum
(transparent layer— protection & barrier)

Stratum granulosum
(granular layer)

Stratum spinosum
(prickle cell layer)

Stratum germinativum
(basal layer—nutrients from dermis & stem cells)

These two layers have nucleus

2. The **dermis** (aka cutis or cutaneous) is a thick layer of skin located beneath the epidermis. It contains dense connective tissue composed mostly of **collagen**. Collagen is largely responsible for the strength of the skin. It allows for the elasticity of skin is noted for. The dermis contains the blood vessels and nerves of the skin and the specialized skin structures of hair follicles and glands. The arrector pili muscles,

which attach to the hair follicles and contract in response to cold and fear, are in the dermis.

The connection between the epidermis and dermis is extremely irregular. It consists of a succession of **papillae** or fingerlike projections. This interlocks the two layers together. The smallest papillae are located where the skin is thinnest (eyelids), and the longest is where the skin is thickest (palms and soles). The papillae of the palms and soles create elevations of the epidermis, which produce ridges. These form fingerprints. Each papilla contains either a capillary loop or a specialized nerve ending. The capillaries supply nutrients to the epidermis. There are four times as many capillaries in the papillae as nerves. The sensory nerve endings give sensations of touch, pain, and temperature, while superficial blood vessels regulate body temperature. The papillae also provide friction that improves our ability to grasp.

3. The **subcutaneous layer** (superficial fascia, subcutis, or hypodermis) is the innermost part of the dermis. It is made up of a layer of fatty tissue called adipose tissue or subcutis, lymph ducts, and blood vessels. The fatty tissue varies

in thickness according to age, sex, and general health. This layer joins the skin to the muscle and other supporting tissues. The adipose tissue provides insulation for the body and protects it from physical shock. The fat can be metabolized to provide the body with energy, and its distribution helps give smoothness to the body and helps determine the male and female body shape. If this tissue becomes hard and loses its elasticity, the layers of skin cannot move properly. Skin elasticity is called skin turgor and can be tested by pinching. The speed at which the skin returns to normal determines the amount of elasticity and hydration.

Note: Some practitioners and histologists consider the subcutaneous tissue as a continuation of the dermis.

Acidity

The skin is slightly acidic: between a pH of 4.8 and 6. This is said to be the acid mantle (mantle – coating or covering). The function of this acid-base is to destroy germs. This protective covering can be destroyed through the use of synthetic soaps, strong preservatives, chemicals found in dyes and other products, washing or bathing in water that is too hot, and stress. It will normally take about 20 minutes to replace the acid mantle once destroyed by a bath.

However, the continued used of substances that either cause build-up in the system or constantly attack the mantle can result in it losing its effectiveness at stopping germs. Many creams, lotions, and washing products damage this acid mantle. While we may look and smell clean, we're open to attack by bacteria and viruses.

The skin has two types of exocrine glands:

1. **Sebaceous glands** (aka oil glands) secrete sebum. They are sac-like glands that lubricate and soften the skin. They normally attach to the hair follicles a short distance below the surface of the epidermis. These glands are the most numerous on the face and scalp. They produce oil for the hair, lubricate the skin, prevent water loss, inhibit the growth of certain types of bacteria, and may destroy some fungi.

2. **Sudoriferous glands** (aka sweat glands) are in the dermis. They are tiny coiled tubes situated in the subcutaneous tissue. From here, a duct extends through the dermis and forms a spiral through the epidermis. Approximately one liter or more of sweat is released per day. These glands extract water, salts, urea, and other waste products and discharge them onto the skin surface as sweat. There are about 3 million, and they are on every part of the body.

Each square inch of skin also contains hundreds of sweat glands. These are controlled by a heat regulation center in the brain. The sweat glands release moisture, which evaporates and cools the body surface (In this capacity, the skin is an excretory organ). Normal body processes produce heat. It is eliminated from the skin by radiation to the surrounding air or by evaporation.

There are two types of sweat glands:
1. **Apocrine sweat glands** are social glands limited to a few regions of the body, primary, auxiliary, and genital areas. Inactive in infants, they develop with puberty and become more active prior to menstruation. Fresh sweat is normally sterile and quite inoffensive. Decomposition by bacteria gives rise to a perspiration odor. (Some believe they play a role in attracting a sexual partner and arousing them sexually).

2. **Exocrine sweat glands** – there are millions of these sweat glands all over the body, and the sweat they give out is little more than diluted saltwater. They help regulate the body to keep its temperature at 98.6 degrees F or 36.8C. These exocrine sweat glands disperse large quantities of water.

Extensions of the Skin

Hair serves as a protective function. The exposed area of the hair is the shaft, and the root is beneath the skin's surface. The root is called the hair follicle. At the bottom of the follicle is a little mound of connective tissue containing capillaries that deliver nutrients to the follicle. Cells multiply at the base, produce keratin, and move outward. They die, and the shaft is composed of dead cells.

Nails or onyx are horny epidermal cells mainly consisting of hard or tough keratin. They are translucent plates that protect the tips of the fingers and toes. The nail plate contains no nerves or blood vessels.

Nerves of the skin:

The skin contains the surface endings of many nerve fibers, such as:

Motor nerve fibers are distributed to the arrector pili muscles attached to the hair follicles. This muscle causes goose flesh when you are frightened or cold.

1. **Sensory nerve fibers** react to heat, cold, touch, pressure, and pain. These sensory receptors send messages to the brain.
2. **Secretory nerve fibers** are distributed to the sweat and oil glands of the skin. These nerves regulate the excretion of perspiration from the sweat glands and control the sebum flow to the skin's surface.

The body replaces over 3 ½ billion cells every day. The skin breathes because it takes in oxygen and discharges carbon dioxide. The skin itself is 50 to 75 percent moisture.

Skin & Body Heat Controls

The skin regulates the temperature of its fatty layers and the internal body through several methods. It does it through the control of heat release and how much heat the body will absorb.

1. **Heat Release Controls.** Temperature is extremely important, as high body temperatures can cause a serious breakdown of the brain and other vital organs. In addition to sweat glands, the major cooling system, 6.5 sq. cm. (one square inch) of skin contains up to 4.5 meters of blood vessels. They help regulate body temperature by **vasoconstriction** (increased

heat retention) and **vasodilatation** (cooling) of blood vessels. When the body temperature rises, vascular dilation allows more blood to flow near the skin's surface. The blood's heat is radiated off. When the temperature is low, blood vessels constrict to reduce blood flow. The less blood near the surface of the skin, the less heat radiated off.

2. **Heat Absorption Controls.** The amount of heat absorbed is a serious problem at times. Sunlight is the main source of external heat that penetrates the body. Heat sources, such as a furnace in a home, do not provide the body heat. It simply allows the skin to feel warm or cool. When sunlight radiation is absorbed to protect the body and skin from too much solar radiation, the skin can increase the production of melanin. This skin color change, most often called tanning, is a skin response to damage caused by radiation. It includes heat absorption. Tanning limits the amount of radiation the skin will absorb.

Nutrition of the Skin

The blood and lymph provide nutrition for the skin. This contributes certain materials for growth, nourishment, skin, hair, and nail repair. Additionally, they remove waste products from the tissues.

Detoxification

The liver and kidneys are considered by most to be the major detoxification organs in the body. However, the skin plays an important role in the detoxification process of the body, not only of itself but of internal organs.

The skin can carry up to 19.8 kilograms (44 lbs) of fat and 9.9 kilograms (22 lbs) of water. This alone ensures that detoxification is essential. The skin can regulate up to 20% of the body's water elimination through perspiration. In this perspiration, urea, uric acid, and other toxins are removed. If the kidneys or liver fail, the skin increases its release of toxins to take the load off the internal organs. Digestive, kidney, intestinal, respiratory, and liver problems frequently indicate their lack of function through the development of skin problems.

Absorption and Penetration of the Skin

Although the skin appears to be a solid barrier, the presence of hair follicles and glands, along with pimples, boils, acne, etc., allow entry of some drugs and chemicals. Many substances cannot enter the skin barrier without a cut or hole. Most artificial substances, such as vitamins, collagen, and elastin, are believed to be unable to cross the skin barrier. Substances that can penetrate the skin include:

- oxygen and carbon dioxide
- fat-soluble vitamins
- hormones (some)
- fat-soluble substances
- gases
- phenol derivatives
- essential oils

Skin Breathing

The skin breathes. It takes in oxygen and discharges carbon dioxide. The amount of carbon dioxide released by the skin in one hour is about 1% of the amount released by the lungs during the same period.

Skin and Water

The skin is 50-75% moisture and can maintain these levels only through sebum. Sebum slows the evaporation of water and limits excess moisture from entering.

The skin can absorb essential oils.

Lymphatic System

Introduction

This is the second type of circulation system, which connects to the blood circulation system. It is often studied as part of the circulatory system; however, as it is the one system stressed in the massage and treatment aspect of aromatherapy, it is considered a separate system in this course.

It consists of circulatory vessels or ducts and nodes. Through these vessels, plasma surrounds and washes the tissue cells and carries out its functions.

Functions

The lymphatic system's main functions include:

1. Production and movement of lymphocytes throughout the body.

2. Drainage of interstitial fluid back into general circulation.

It also has a number of secondary functions that are the result of the two main ones.
They are:

- The removal of toxic wastes.
- The resistance to or fighting disease.
- The nourishment of tissue cells.
- The movement of digested fat from the intestine to the bloodstream

Lymph

Lymph is the fluid carried in the lymphatic system. Lymph is simply plasma that has excluded or oozed from the capillaries. It contains a large number of white blood cells. Lymph is medically classified as fluid tissue due to its number of living cells.

Lymph is a transparent, usually slightly yellow, often opalescent liquid. It is about 95% water, with the rest comprising plasma proteins and other chemical substances in blood plasma. Usually, the percentage is slightly smaller than in plasma. Its cellular component consists chiefly of lymphocytes.

The body contains three main fluids: blood, tissue, and lymph. When the plasma, without solid particles, seeps through the capillary walls and circulates among the body tissues, it is called tissue fluid. When this fluid is drained from the tissues and collected by the lymphatic system, it is known as lymph. The plasma nourishes the cells, and the tissue fluid assists with removing waste from the cells. It then diffuses into the lymphatic capillaries from the space between the cells. This space is known as the interstice. The fluid filling this space is called interstitial fluid.

The synovial fluid that lubricates joints is almost identical to lymph. The serous fluid found in the body and pleural cavities is also not lymph, although it is very similar. The fluid contained within the ear's semicircular canals, known as endolymph, is not lymph.

Muscular System

Introduction

Where the skeletal system is the foundation of our bodies, the muscular system is the framing. It provides not only strength but it helps to hold the foundation together. These two systems are closely related, as any problems with the skeletal system will most likely be noticed in the muscular system.

Physiology

The muscular system is made up of 640 named muscles in the body and thousands of unnamed ones. Muscles are responsible for up to 50% of the total body weight. Muscle tissue is an organ characterized by its ability to contract. The contraction is usually in response to a stimulus the nervous system provides.

Function

Their primary function is to permit movement to the skeleton. This movement is achieved through the muscles pulling against the leverage the bones and their joints provide.

Muscle Types

There are three types of muscle:

1. Voluntary (aka Skeletal Muscle): They operate under our conscious control. Skeletal muscle consists of long fibers surrounded by a sheath. These fibers are elongated sausage-shaped cells. The cells exhibit striation (grooves or ridges) that look like individual fibers in the muscle. Voluntary muscles are striated. The nerves that supply the muscle are from the central nervous system. Voluntary muscle is the meat of animals and is responsible for skeletal movement. These muscles can provide sudden bursts of energy or strength, but only for a short period.

2. Involuntary (aka Smooth Muscle): They are not under our conscious control. They are responsible for the life-preserving functions of the body. They are sometimes called visceral or smooth muscles. The muscle is composed of spindle-shaped cells. The muscle has no cross striations but may have faint longitudinal striations. Involuntary muscles are smooth. The autonomic nervous

system stimulates the muscle. Smooth muscle is located in the skin, internal organs, reproductive system, major blood vessels, and the excretory system. These muscles have the capability of working for long periods; however, they do not have the capability of providing sudden bursts of energy.

3. Cardiac Muscle: This muscle is composed of mostly involuntary muscle fiber but bears a superficial resemblance to voluntary muscle in that there is some poorly defined striation. It makes up most of the heart and is found only in the heart. Cardiac muscle is normally outside conscious control. It can be, however, affected by conscious thought. The nerves from the autonomic nervous system speed or slow its action.

Neurological System

Introduction

The neurological or nervous system consists of structures concerned with receiving stimuli from internal or external receptors, transmitting nerve impulses to and from the brain, or activating muscle mechanisms.

Contrary to popular belief, it is not simply an electrical system. It is based on an electrical-chemical function. All protoplasm is excitable and conductive. (Protoplasm is the semi-fluid translucent substance that constitutes the living matter of cells and includes the nucleus and cytoplasm.) Nerve cells or neurons are only one cell type but are especially excitable and sensitive. They are specialized fibers designed to rapidly move impulses throughout their length and onto the next cell.

The nervous system is a network found throughout the body. It provides two-way communication and a coordinated response to any stimulus. Most think of the system as a series of long nerves reaching from the brain to specific locations in the body made up of one long continuous fiber. In fact, the nerve is made up of thousands of individual cells. Between each cell is a very small gap called a synapse. The electric impulse moves through the cell and causes a chemical reaction that carries the impulse across the gap and initiates the electrical impulse in the next nerve cell.

Function

The function of the nervous system is to relay information in the form of nerve impulses throughout the body, thereby controlling all its functions.

System Divisions

The neurological system has two main divisions. They are the:

1.   Central Nervous System (CNS) comprises the brain and spinal column. This is referred to as cerebrospinal.

2.   Peripheral Nervous System (PNS) - includes all neural structures outside the CNS. (Sense organs, muscles, and glands) It is made up of 12 pairs of cranial nerves and 31 pairs of spinal nerves.

It is divided into two parts or divisions, the somatic and the autonomic. They work as follows:

1. Somatic is composed of nerve receptors that are concerned with changes outside the body. *Stimulus*

2. Autonomic is concerned with the regulation of the internal environment. *Response.* (Sympathetic and parasympathetic)

Something Interesting for Your Mind

Read the note below... You'll be amazed...

The paomnnehil pweor of the hmuan mnid. Aoccrdnig to a rscheearch at Cmabrigde Uinervtisy, it deosn't mttaer in waht oredr the ltteers in a wrod are, the olny iprmoetnt tinhg is taht the fist and lsat ltteer be at the rghit pclae. The rset can be a taotl mses and you can sitll raed it wouthit porbelm. This is bcuseae the huanm mnid deos not raed ervey lteter by istlef, but the wrod as a wlohe.

AMZANIG HUH?

Reproductive System

The Female

Introduction

The reproductive system is one of the body's systems that varies by sex. Although separate and distinct, the two systems are, in fact, closely aligned.

The male and female reproductive systems consist of organs and glands that belong to or carry out both endocrine and reproductive functions. This section will concentrate on reproductive functions.

Female Reproductive System
The function of the female reproductive system is to:

- Produce ovum
- Produce offspring

The primary parts of the female reproductive system consist of:

- Ovaries (2)
- Fallopian Tubes (Uterine Tubes or Oviducts) (2)
- Uterus

- Vagina
- Vulva
- Breasts

The Male

Introduction

The male reproductive system has often been considered less complicated than the female one. That concept is changing as an understanding of male health and its impact on fertility is developed.

Male Reproductive System

The function of the male reproductive system is to:

- Produce sperm
- Fertilize the ovum

The primary parts of the male reproductive system consist of the:

- Testis (testes/testicles)
- Spermatic Cord
- Vas deferens

- Cowper's Gland
- Prostate Gland
- Penis
- Scrotum

Respiratory System

Introduction

The respiratory system is a close partner to the cardiovascular system. They both provide oxygen to the body and remove carbon dioxide and other waste products. It is also one of the most open systems. It brings in a wide variety of things, from dust to viruses, with the air and is susceptible to injury and disease.

Respiration

Respiration means 'breathe again.' Respiration is a physical process by which living organisms take oxygen from the surrounding medium and emit carbon dioxide. The respiratory system carries out respiration for the body.

Functions

- The respiratory system is responsible for the following specific functions:
- Oxygen-carbon dioxide exchange via inspiration and expiration

- maintaining proper acid-base balance in the blood
- speech production.

Structure of the Respiratory System

The respiratory tract is normally divided into:
- the upper respiratory tract allows airflow in and out of the lungs.
- the lower respiratory tract, which allows for gas exchange at the alveoli level.

Skeletal System

Introduction

The skeletal system is composed of the bones in our body. It is the foundation of the body, and its health plays an important role in the overall health of the body.

Physiology

The skeleton has several functions. It provides the framework for the body as well as a place for muscles to attach. The organs and glands are held in place by attachments directly or indirectly to the bone. The bones also produce red blood cells in the bone marrow.

The main bone functions are:

- **PROTECTION.** The ribs protect the heart and lungs.
- **LOCOMOTION.** The skeleton allows movement by providing a fulcrum or lever for the muscles to pull against. This, in turn, causes movement.
- **PRODUCTION OF RED AND WHITE BLOOD CELLS BY BONE MARROW.**
- **STORAGE OF MINERALS SUCH AS CALCIUM AND PHOSPHOROUS**

Urinary System

Introduction

The urinary system is, of course, closely linked and positioned to the reproductive organs. In the male, the urethra has shared responsibility with both the reproductive and urinary systems. This is a very simple system, yet it plays a very important role in maintaining homeostasis in the body.

System Parts

The excretory organs and parts consist of:

- Kidneys
- Ureters
- Bladder
- Urethra

Waste Production

The principle metabolic wastes are water, carbon dioxide, and wastes that contain nitrogen. Amino acids contain nitrogen.

The nitrogen-containing amino group is removed when they are broken down in the liver. The amino group is then converted to ammonia and then to urea. Also, the nucleic acid is broken down to form uric acid. These are transported from the liver to the kidneys by the blood.

TCRS ESO For Each System Of The Body

	Top	Middle	Base
Cardiovascular	Ravensara	Lavender	
Circulation	Aniseed Clary Sage Eucalyptus Lemon Lime Lista Cubeba Mandarin Orange(all) Thyme Yarrow Cardamom	Black Pepper Chamomile Geranium Juniper Berry Lavandin Lavender Melissa Peppermint Pine Rosemary Sage Spruce	Benzoin Cedarwood Linden Blossom Neroli Nutmeg Rose Tarragon Vetiver Ylang Ylang Ginger
Digestive	Aniseed Basil Bay Bergamot Clary Sage Coriander (seed) Grapefruit Lemon Lemongrass Lime Lista Cubeba Mandarin	Black Pepper Camphor(white) Fennel(sweet) Hyssop Juniper Berry Lavender Manuka Marjoram Peppermint Rosemary Sage	Clove Frankincense Ginger Immortelle Myrrh Neroli Nutmeg Patchouli Spikenard Tarragon

	Orange (sweet) Orange (bitter) Palmarosa Spearmint Thyme Yarrow Verbena		
Endocrine	Mandarin Palmarosa	Geranium Lavender Pine	Jasmine Neroli Rose Vetiver Ylang Ylang
Genital/Urinary	Basil Bay Bergamot Cardamom Clary Sage Niaouli Orange (blood) Tea Tree	Black Pepper Cypress Fennel (sweet) Geranium Juniper Manuka Sage	Cedarwood (all) Frankincense Jasmine Myrrh Rose Sandalwood
Immune	Aniseed Bay Cajeput Coriander Eucalyptus Lemon Lemongrass Lime Orange (bitter/blood) Petitgrain	Fir Hyssop Lavender Manuka Melissa Rosewood Sage Spruce	Nutmeg

	Ravensara Tea Tree Thyme Yarrow		
Lymph	Grapefruit	Fennel(sweet) Chamomile Cypress Juniper Lavender	Ginger Immortelle
Muscles	Basil Bay Bergamot Cajeput Cardamom Eucalyptus Lemongrass Niaouli Orange(all) Petitgrain Thyme Yarrow	Black Pepper Camphor Chamomile Fir Lavandin Lavender Marjoram Melissa Myrtle Peppermint Rosemary Rosewood Sage Spruce	Cedarwood Jasmine Nutmeg Patchouli Sandalwood Tarragon Vetiver Ylang Ylang
Nerves	Basil Bergamot Cardamom Clary Sage Coriander(seed) Grapefruit Lemongrass Mandarin Orange(sweet) Palmarosa Tea Tree Verbena	Camphor (white) Fir Geranium Lavandin Lavender Lavender(spike) Marjoram Melissa Spruce	Benzoin Cedarwood Clove Frankincense Immortelle Jasmine Linden Blossom Nutmeg Neroli Patchouli Tarragon Vetiver Ylang Ylang

Reproductive	Aniseed Lista Cubeba Palmarosa Verbena	Hyssop Lavender	Spikenard Tarragon
Respiratory	Aniseed Basil Cajeput Clary Sage Coriander Eucalyptus Lemon Lime Litsea Cubeba Tea Tree Thyme	Camphor (white) Cypress Fir Hyssop Lavender Manuka Marjoram Peppermint Pine Rosemary	Benzoin Cedarwood Clove Frankincense Immortelle Myrrh Linden Blossom Sandalwood
Skin	Bergamot Eucalyptus Grapefruit Lemon Lemongrass Lime Litsea Cubeba Mandarin Niaouli Orange (all) Palmarosa Petitgrain Ravensara Tea Tree	Camphor (white) Chamomile Fennel(sweet) Geranium Hyssop Juniper Lavandin Lavender (spike) Manuka Myrrh Myrtle Pine Rosewood	Benzoin Cedarwood Frankincense Ginger Immortelle Jasmine Linden Blossom Myrrh Neroli Patchouli Rose Spikenard Vetiver Ylang Ylang
Skeletal	Cajeput	Black Pepper Lavender Myrtle	Clove

How Essential Oils are Tested for Quality

There are a number of methods to test the quality of essential oil; the essential oil quality tests attempt to determine the components of the essential oil and if any suspicious elements have been added or removed; the quality tests for essential oils include:

- ➢ Gas Liquid Chromatography (GLC)
- ➢ Mass Spectrometry (GC-MS)
- ➢ Optical Rotation
- ➢ Infrared Test
- ➢ Refractive Index

GAS LIQUID CHROMATOGRAPHY

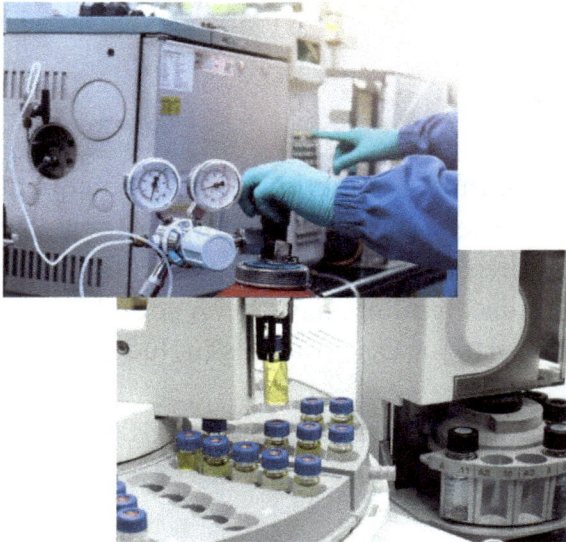

AKA, Gas Chromatography is used in analytical chemistry for separating and analyzing compounds – specifically, gas-liquid chromatography - involves a sample being vaporized and injected onto the head of the chromatographic column.

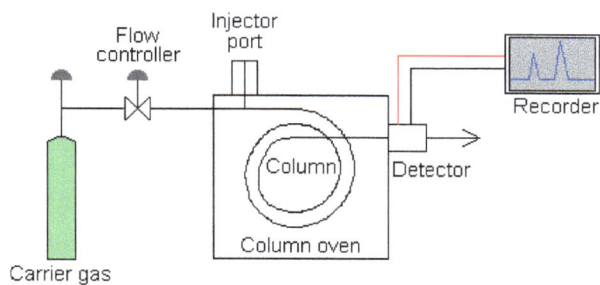

The sample is transported through the column by the flow of inert, gaseous mobile phase and is read by the recorder.

MASS SPECTROMETRY QUALITY TEST

The Mass Spectrometry quality test is a more expensive test for essential oil quality; gas chromatography-mass spectrometry (GC-MS) is an advanced version of the gas-liquid chromatography quality test. An essential oil supplier may be able to provide the reports of the GC-MS analysis of essential oil to demonstrate the quality and purity of the essential oils supplied.

The mass spectrometer is attached to the gas chromatograph, and the emerging essential oil molecules are hit with high-energy electrons to separate them. GC-MS testing separates the individual components of the essential oil and allows the identification of each chemical component by comparison to the molecular mass spectrum of the essential oil.

Examples from New Directions Aromatics (2010)

New Directions
AROMATICS

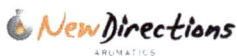

GC ANALYSIS – ANISEED ESSENTIAL OIL

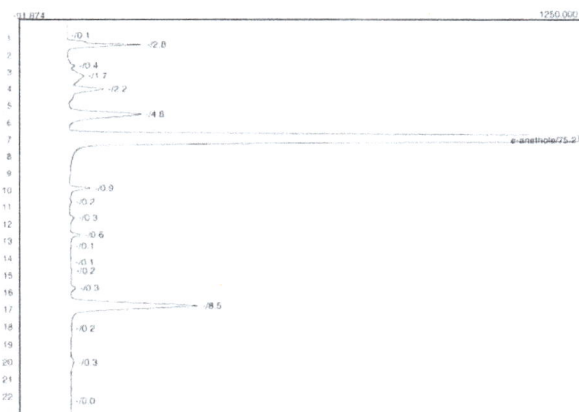

Preparation Information:
Quality Assurance
New Directions Aromatics Inc.

Date Revised: March 2007

Disclaimer

The information contained in this GC Analysis is obtained using our own equipment. However, as the ordinary or otherwise use(s) of this product is outside the control of New Directions Aromatics Inc., no representation or warranty, expressed or implied, is made as to the effect(s) of such use(s) (including damage or injury) or the results obtained.

New Directions Aromatics Inc. expressly disclaims responsibility as to the ordinary or otherwise use(s) of this product. As to the fitness for any use, New Directions Aromatics will not make any recommendations; nothing on our website or associated documentation should be considered as such. The liability of New Directions Aromatics Inc. is limited to the value of the goods, and does not include any consequential loss.

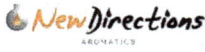

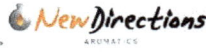

New Directions
AROMATICS
<!--[if !vml]-->
[endif]-->

New Directions
AROMATICS
<!--

GC ANALYSIS – CEDARWOOD VIRGINIAN ESSENTIAL OIL

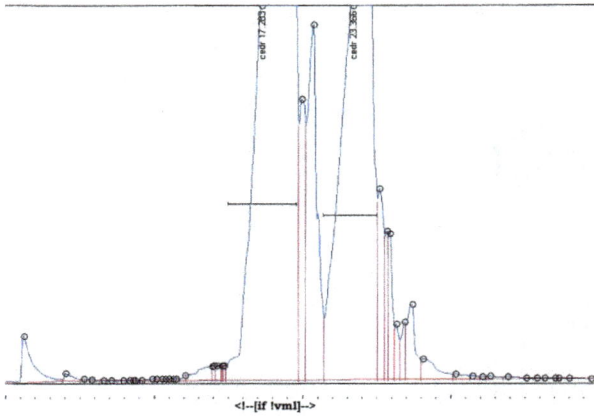

<!--[if !vml]-->

New Directions
AROMATICS

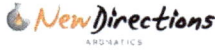

GC ANALYSIS – GERANIUM EGYPTIAN ESSENTIAL OIL

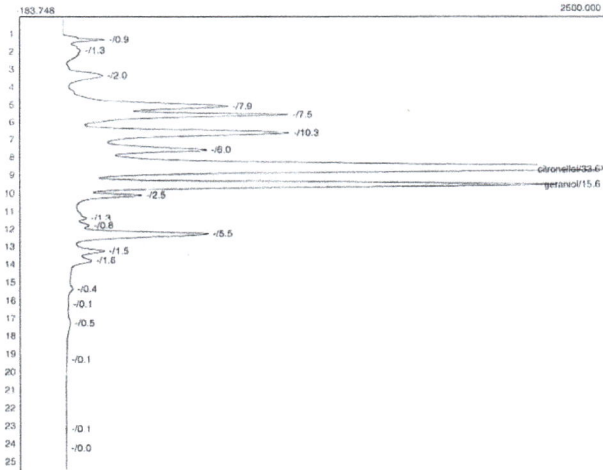

183.748		2500.000

```
1        -/0.9
2        -/1.3
3        -/2.0
4
5              -/7.9        -/7.5
6                           -/10.3
7        -/6.0
8
9                                    citronellol/33.6
10       -/2.5                       geraniol/15.6
11       -/1.3
12       -/0.8        -/5.5
13       -/1.5
14       -/1.6
15       -/0.4
16       -/0.1
17       -/0.5
18
19       -/0.1
20
21
22
23       -/0.1
24       -/0.0
25
```

Preparation Information:
Quality Assurance
New Directions Aromatics Inc.

Date Revised: June 2007

Disclaimer

The information contained in this GC Analysis is obtained using our own equipment. However, as the ordinary or otherwise use(s) of this product is outside the control of New Directions Aromatics Inc., no representation or warranty, expressed or implied, is made as to the effect (s) of such use(s) (including damage or injury) or the results obtained.

New Directions Aromatics Inc. expressly disclaims responsibility as to the ordinary or otherwise use(s) of this product. As to the fitness for any use, New Directions Aromatics will not make any recommendations; nothing on our website or associated documentation should be considered as such. The liability of New Directions Aromatics Inc. is limited to the value of the goods, and does not include any consequential loss.

Report the retention time of each peak (in minutes) = time it takes the molecule to be identified by the chromatograph.

Area = (height) x (width at ½ height)
Mark retention time, height, half-height, and width at ½ height

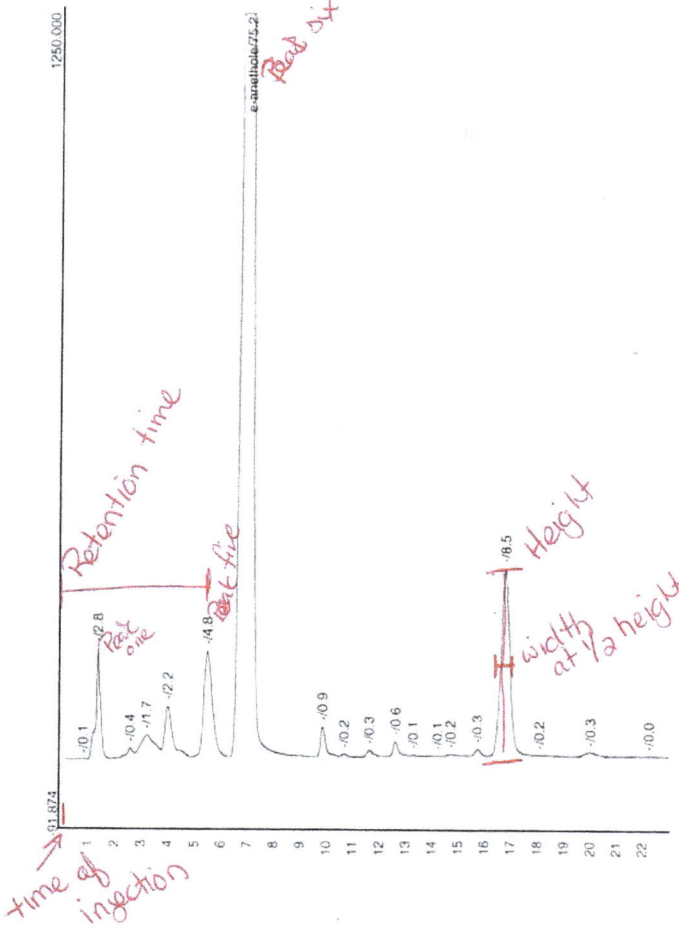

Optical Rotation

Optical rotation, also known as polarization rotation or circular birefringence, is the rotation of the orientation of the plane of polarization about the optical axis of linearly polarized light as it travels through certain materials. Circular birefringence and circular dichroism are the manifestations of optical activity.

Infrared Test

Infrared Spectroscopy: Chemical Composition and Identification of Polymers and Organic Compounds

FT-IR, Fourier Transform Infrared Spectroscopy, is an exceptional means for the profiling and screening sample compounds. It is used to identify the chemical compounds in a wide range of products, including coatings, foods, paints, pharmaceuticals, consumer products, and polymers, to name a few. FT Infrared Spectroscopy is a useful analytical device for the detection of functional groups and for describing covalent bonding data.

Refractive Index

In optics, a material's refractive index (also known as refraction index or index of refraction) is a dimensionless number that describes how fast light travels through the material.

Time of Harvest!!!

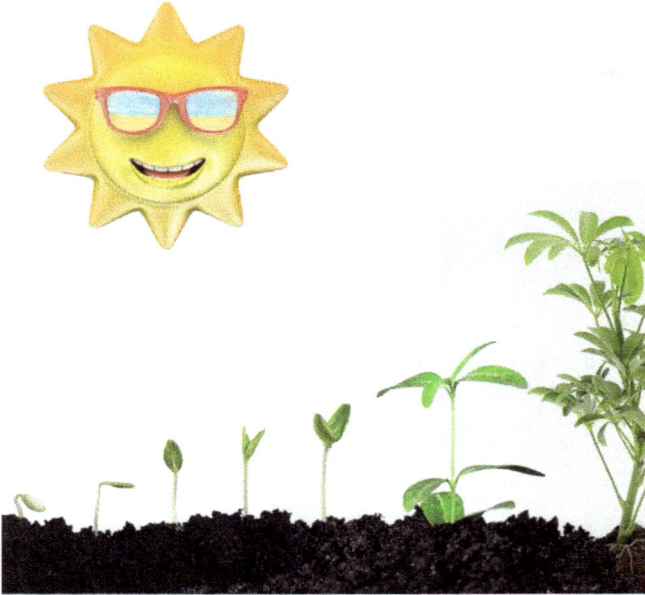

Did you know that the time of harvest affects the percentage and proportions of various chemical constituents in the plant? Therefore, the oil quality will differ depending on when the plant is harvested. Was it just sprouted, fully grown, or somewhere in between?

Also, what part of the plant is used will make a difference in the chemical constituents (roots, stems, leaves, flowers, or fruit).

Bark
>Cassia, Cinnamon

Berries/Fruit
>Black Pepper, Juniper Berry,
>May Chang (Litsea Cubeba)

Citrus Rinds
>Bergamot, Grapefruit, Lemon, Lime, Mandarin,
>Orange, Tangerine

Flowering Herbs
>(Typical Distillation of Both Flowers and Leaves)
>Basil, Clary Sage, Hyssop, Lavender, Lavendin,
>Lemon Balm (Melissa), Marjoram, Oregano,
>Peppermint, Rosemary, Sage, Spearmint, Thyme,
>Yarrow

Flowers/Petals/Buds
>Boronia, Chamomile (all), Clove, Helichrysum,
>Jasmine, Linden Blossom, Neroli, Rose,
>Tuberose, Ylang Ylang

Grass
>Citronella, Lemongrass, Palmarosa

Leaves

Bay, Bergamot, Cajeput, Cinnamon, Eucalyptus, Geranium, Lemon Myrtle, Manuka, Myrtle, Niaouli, Patchouli, Petitgrain, Ravensara, Tea Tree, Violet

Moss/Lichen

Oakmoss

Needles

Cypress, Fir, Scotch Pine, Spruce

Resin/Balsam/Gum

Benzoin, Balsam, Elemi, Frankincense, Myrrh

Roots

Angelica, Ginger, Spikenard, Vetiver

Seeds

Ambrette, Anise, Cardamom, Carrot, Coriander, Cumin, Dill, Fennel, Nutmeg,

Wood

Amyris, Cedarwood (all), Rosewood, Sandalwood

And some essential oils are derived from multiple parts of the botanical.

- Cinnamon bark or leaf
- Clove bud or leaf

It is helpful to know what part(s) of a plant was used in the production of essential oil, as the constituents, aroma, safety precautions, and therapeutic properties of the essential oil can vary.

Different species will have different percentages and proportions of various chemical constituents.

E.g., Lavender

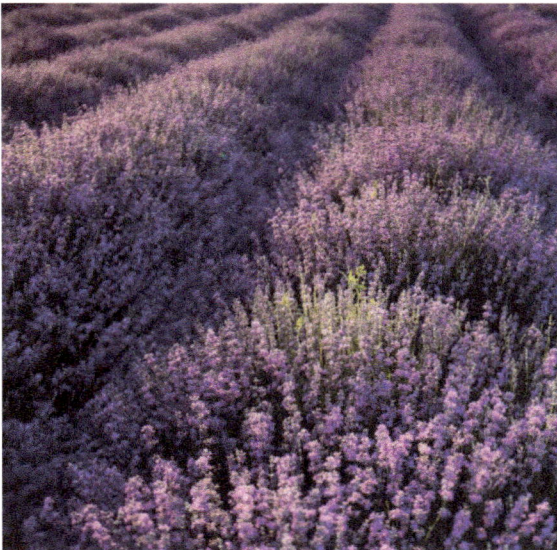

Lavender is a flowering shrub in the Lamiaceae (mint) family and boasts over 40 known species with an ever-growing count of over 400 cultivated varieties. While it is native to areas near the Mediterranean, Lavender is now grown worldwide, and the various species provide us with several different essential oils.

Part of the plant used: Flowers
Family: Lamiaceae
Genus: Lavandula
Species:

- L. angustifolia,
- L. spica,
- L. spicata,
- L. stoechas,
- L. x intermedia,
- L. officinalis,
- L. vera,
- L. latifolia.

Common names:
English lavender, French lavender, lavandin, Spanish lavender, high altitude lavender, Himalayan lavender, lavender mailette, population lavender, lavender fine, spike lavender, lavandin grosso, lavandin super, lavandin abrial, Bulgarian lavender.

Dominant chemical constituents:
Linalool, linalyl acetate, 1,8 cineole, camphor, (lavandulyl acetate, lavandulol, terpinene-4-ol, beta-caryophyllene).

Therapeutic properties:
Emotionally calming, support the respiratory system, skin-regenerating, pain-relieving, antispasmodic, anti-inflammatory, antimicrobial.

Lavenders are well known for having high linalool, a monoterpenol, content. What makes Lavandula angustifolia different is that it contains a high percentage of esters, particularly linalyl acetate. This monoterpenol-ester synergy is what characterizes *Lavandula angustifolia*.

Lavandula angustifolia, formerly known as L. officinalis or L. vera, is the lavender you will purchase most often and which is the most commonly available. It is primarily grown in Europe and maybe named true lavender, Bulgarian lavender, English lavender, high altitude lavender, Himalayan lavender, lavender Kashmir, lavender maillette, or any of several other names.

L. angustifolia plants produce less essential oil than the hybrid Lavandin plants do. 6 to 8 plants' worth of *L. angustifolia* flowering stalks will fill the basket of a 15-gallon copper alembic still and will yield about 70ml of essential oil per distillation.

L. angustifolia has the calming effect of the esters in the monoterpenol-ester synergy, making it the go-to for soothing and calming anxious or busy thoughts, soothing symptoms that are related to stress (headache, occasional sleeplessness, restlessness, nausea, agitation, etc.), and helping the body to relax. *The biggest difference among these various *L. angustifolia* varieties is where the lavender is grown.

Compare it to *L. latifolia*, or spike lavender, with expectorant and mucolytic properties. It is an excellent choice for respiratory support and to address headache pain. It is also a good choice in cases of skin damage (burns, cuts, scrapes, stings, etc.), especially where antimicrobial support is desired. It supports the musculoskeletal system and can be used in case of muscle or joint pain.

Interesting Fact

A pure essential oil will, by its very nature, will have natural chemical differences between batches of the same essential oil due to a number of factors, **including climate, soil, the country in which the plant was grown, and the altitude at which the plant was grown before the essential oil was extracted.**

The action of any complete oil cannot be forecast with accuracy only on the basis of individual constituents. Some components modify others. There is a direct relationship between a chemical arrangement and therapeutic properties, but it is very complex.

To understand the importance of the chemical constituents in the plant, we must go back to the basics.

Essential oils are mixtures of aromatic molecules produced from three basic elements: carbon, hydrogen, and oxygen.

Chemical Components of an Essential Oil

Chemical Structure

ATOM

The atom was once believed to be the smallest object in existence. It is the basic building block of the universe.

Atoms are composed of a nucleus containing one or more protons, which have an electrically positive charge, and one or more neutrons, which are neutral and contain one positive and one negative charge. Circling around the nucleus are orbits or shells containing electrons, which are negatively charged particles. Generally, the atoms require two electrons in the innermost orbit or shell and eight in all other further orbits. The number of orbits depends on the number of protons in the nucleus of each individual atom. These values are conventionally agreed upon and set in the chemical periodic table. The atomic number refers to the number of protons in an atom. It is equal to the number of electrons circling the nucleus in a neutral atom.

The atomic weight is a unit of measurement describing the weight of the atomic nucleus. Atoms often are unsaturated. They lack the correct number of electrons and need to join other atoms to gain the number they need to be in balance or saturated.

An atom consists of an electron(s) and nucleus (neutron, proton, and quark):

Nucleus: Center of something – Atom nucleus, made up of positively charged protons and neutral neutrons.

Neutron: A subatomic particle with no electric charge.

Proton: A baryon comprises two up quarks and one down quark.

Quark: Building blocks of protons and neutrons.

Atom

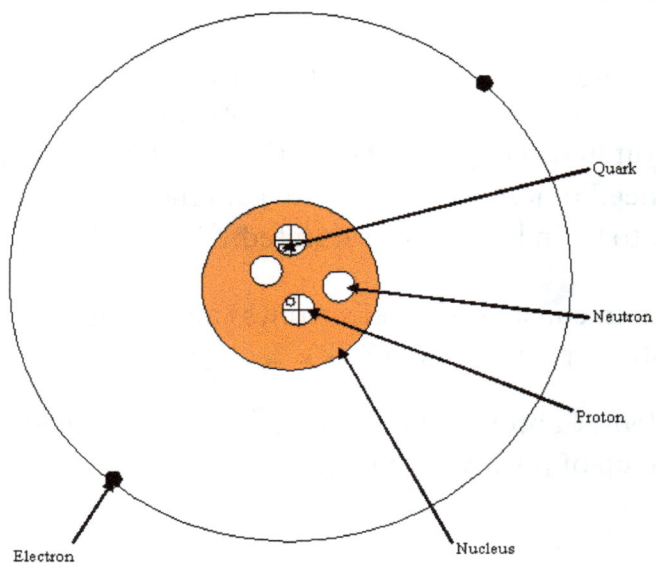

Electron: An elementary particle that carries a negative charge. These electrons zoom around the nucleus in a 3D orbit called a shell (there can be many shells in an electron cloud).

> *The first* shell has up to 2 electrons
> *Second and third* have up to 8
> *Fourth and fifth* have up to 18
> *Sixth* has up to 32

The Periodic Table shows all the atomic numbers; this tells the number of protons in an atom, which always equals the number of electrons.

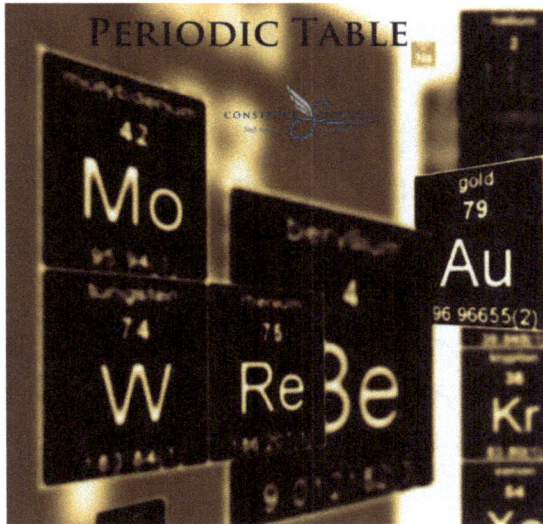

Hydrogen atom

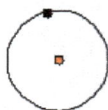

Helium atom

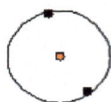

Lithium atom

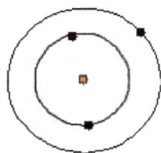

Berylium atom

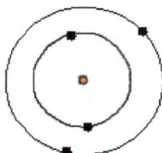

Draw in the appropriate number of electrons:

Neon element

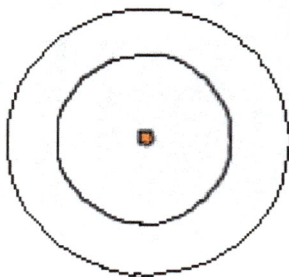

Atomic Mass _____
Number of Protons _____
Number of Electrons _____

Sulphur element

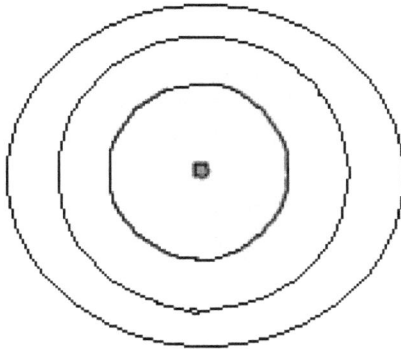

Atomic Mass _____
Number of Protons _____
Number of Electrons _____

ELEMENTS

A chemical element (element) is a substance consisting
of chemically identical atoms that cannot be
decomposed or transformed into any other chemical
substance by ordinary chemical processes.

Periodic Table of Elements

Legend (example):

14
Si
Silicon
28.1

Atomic Number
Symbol
Name
Atomic Mass

1	2	3	4	5	6	7	8	9	10	11	12	13	14	15	16	17	18
1 H Hydrogen 1.0																	2 He Helium 4.0
3 Li Lithium 6.9	4 Be Beryllium 9.0											5 B Boron 10.8	6 C Carbon 12.0	7 N Nitrogen 14.0	8 O Oxygen 16.0	9 F Fluorine 19.0	10 Ne Neon 20.2
11 Na Sodium 23.0	12 Mg Magnesium 24.3											13 Al Aluminium 27.0	14 Si Silicon 28.1	15 P Phosphorus 31.0	16 S Sulphur 32.1	17 Cl Chlorine 35.5	18 Ar Argon 39.9
19 K Potassium 39.1	20 Ca Calcium 40.1	21 Sc Scandium 45.0	22 Ti Titanium 47.9	23 V Vanadium 50.9	24 Cr Chromium 52.0	25 Mn Manganese 54.9	26 Fe Iron 55.8	27 Co Cobalt 58.9	28 Ni Nickel 58.7	29 Cu Copper 63.5	30 Zn Zinc 65.4	31 Ga Gallium 69.7	32 Ge Germanium 72.6	33 As Arsenic 74.9	34 Se Selenium 79.0	35 Br Bromine 79.9	36 Kr Krypton 83.8
37 Rb Rubidium 85.5	38 Sr Strontium 87.6	39 Y Yttrium 88.9	40 Zr Zirconium 91.2	41 Nb Niobium 92.9	42 Mo Molybdenum 95.9	43 Tc Technetium 98	44 Ru Ruthenium 101.1	45 Rh Rhodium 102.9	46 Pd Palladium 106.4	47 Ag Silver 107.9	48 Cd Cadmium 112.4	49 In Indium 114.8	50 Sn Tin 118.7	51 Sb Antimony 121.8	52 Te Tellurium 127.6	53 I Iodine 126.9	54 Xe Xenon 131.3
55 Cs Cesium 132.9	56 Ba Barium 137.3	57 La Lanthanum 138.9	72 Hf Hafnium 178.5	73 Ta Tantalum 180.9	74 W Tungsten 183.8	75 Re Rhenium 186.2	76 Os Osmium 190.2	77 Ir Iridium 192.2	78 Pt Platinum 195.1	79 Au Gold 197.0	80 Hg Mercury 200.6	81 Tl Thallium 204.4	82 Pb Lead 207.2	83 Bi Bismuth 209.0	84 Po Polonium 209	85 At Astatine 210	86 Rn Radon 222
87 Fr Francium 223	88 Ra Radium 226	89 Ac Actinium 227	104 Rf Rutherfordium 261	105 Db Dubnium 262	106 Sg Seaborgium 263	107 Bh Bohrium 262	108 Hs Hassium 265	109 Mt Meitnerium 266									

58 Ce Cerium 140.1	59 Pr Praseodymium 140.9	60 Nd Neodymium 144.2	61 Pm Promethium 145	62 Sm Samarium 150.4	63 Eu Europium 152.0	64 Gd Gadolinium 157.3	65 Tb Terbium 158.9	66 Dy Dysprosium 162.5	67 Ho Holmium 164.9	68 Er Erbium 167.3	69 Tm Thulium 168.9	70 Yb Ytterbium 173.0	71 Lu Lutetium 175.0
90 Th Thorium 232.0	91 Pa Protactinium 231.0	92 U Uranium 238.0	93 Np Neptunium 237	94 Pu Plutonium 244	95 Am Americium 243	96 Cm Curium 247	97 Bk Berkelium 247	98 Cf Californium 251	99 Es Einsteinium 252	100 Fm Fermium 257	101 Md Mendelevium 258	102 No Nobelium 259	103 Lr Lawrencium 262

Based on mass of C12 at 12.00.
Values in Parentheses are the masses of the most stable or best known isotopes for elements which do not occur naturally.

Element	Abbreviation	% in the body	Important For
Calcium	Ca	2	Tone, power, strength. Stored in bone and teeth also helps growth and maintain them. Calms nerves, iron absorption, brain concentration, heart regulation and happiness.
Carbon (*Black ball)	C	18	Everything alive has carbon elements.
Chlorine	Cl	.15	Cleanse- fights germs and bacteria, Liver detoxifier, Helps digestion, joints and tendons. Balances liquid and electrolytes.
Hydrogen (*White ball)	H	10	Life itself
Iodine	I	trace	Improves all organ function. Helps burn fat, Very important to the brain (alertness), thyroid (growth), spleen and liver (toxins). Healing of sores and ulcers.

Iron	Fe	.004	Hemoglobin (red blood cells). Improves mind, stress, self-esteem, and energy levels. Aids in transporting oxygen. Aids in preventing colds.
Magnesium	Mg	.05	Relaxation, Digestion (enzymes, carbohydrates, amino, other minerals and blood sugar to blood). Improves sleep. Strengthens teeth and bones. Needed for lungs, brain, cardiovascular and neuromuscular contractions.
Manganese	Mn	trace	CNS, memory, intelligence, reflexes, calmness, sight, sex hormone, pituitary and thyroid. Blood sugar levels and fertility
Nitrogen (*Blue ball)	N	3	With carbon process protein
Oxygen (*Red ball)	O	65	Vital for functioning of blood cells
Phosphorous (*Purple ball)	P	1	Brain (intelligence), energy level, bone & teeth, heartbeat,

			kidney function, reproduction, burns carbohydrates, fats and protein. Emotional -caring
Potassium	K	.35	Muscle building, adrenal glands, elimination, heartbeat, fluid balance, blood sugar, hair, nerves, skin elasticity and vitality.
Sodium	Na	.15	Active and limber, Acid/Alkaline balance, elimination of carbon dioxide, liver, pancreas, spleen, digestion, muscles, nerves, fluids, organs and connective tissue. Prevention of blood clotting and improves osmosis.
Sulphur (*Yellow ball)	S	.25	Active, brain, nerves, liver, skin detoxifier, fights bacterial infections, collagen and homeostasis.
Zinc	Zn	trace	Mind, sex organs, DNA, T cells, growth, vitamin absorption, carbohydrate, phosphorus balance, enzyme, insulin &

			healing of wounds and burns.

Are the colors of the plastic elemental build spheres (balls) used to demo organic molecules?

Hydrogen is a diatomic element; it always has a bond of two atoms and Nitrogen, Oxygen, Fluorine, Chlorine, Bromine, and Iodine in the periodic table. All other elements can exist alone.

Abbreviations

When referring to elements in chemistry, the first letter capitalized is used to depict the element. An example would be hydrogen or H and carbon or C.

ION

This is an electrically charged atom or group of atoms. An example would be Na+ Cl-. Elements are either positive or negatively charged, depending on their number of protons or electrons. More electrons in the shell than protons in the nuclei make the element negative, and more protons in the nuclei than electrons in the shell make the element positive.

All elements that are metals are positive (cations), and nonmetals are all negative (anions). Metals bond only with nonmetals (ionic bonds), and nonmetals can bond with either metals or each other (covalent bonds).

MOLECULES

A molecule is the **smallest part of an element or compound that can exist alone.** It is formed when two or more atoms join together. The combinations of atoms form complex molecules. The combination of molecules results in the formation of all chemicals and objects. They can be the same element or different elements.

- The hydrogen molecule is H2, two of the same elements.
- The oxygen molecule is O2, also two of the same elements.

For interest sake, in one drop of essential oil, there are 40,000,000,000,000.000,000,000 (40 sextillions) or forty thousand million, million, million molecules. On the cellular scale, therefore, amounts of chemicals, which seem insignificant, can, in fact, be very significant.

Carbon atoms can join with other carbon atoms to form chains or rings. With the addition of each atom, the resulting molecule gets heavier and heavier. So, as an example, the lighter one-carbon or methane molecule (CH4) becomes the heavier propane molecule (C3H8) with the addition of 2 carbon and 4 hydrogen atoms.

COMPOUNDS

Is a substance consisting of elements combined in fixed and defined proportions by weight? An example would be CO2.

Water is H2O, two different elements, but it can be broken down into hydrogen and oxygen.
Oxygenating compounds lend the greatest potential of increasing oxygen in support of the immune function.

CONSTITUENT(S)

This is one or more chemical(s) that make up the essential oil.

BONDS

A bond is the connecting of atoms to share electrons. Examples of the three atoms that share electrons to bond to make up essential oils:

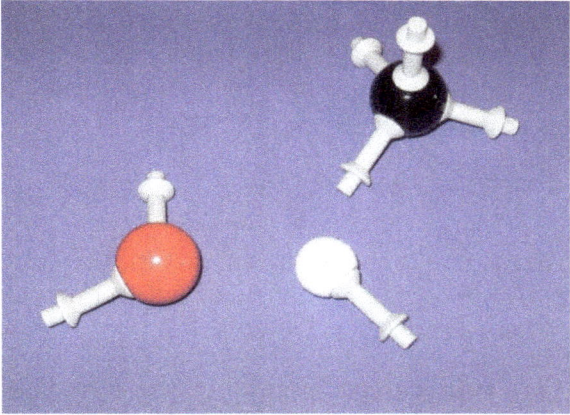

- Carbon (black ball) has six electrons, meaning it can either gain four electrons to complete the *second* electron shell or give four electrons to complete the *first* electron shell. Either way, it has to have four electrons to bond with other elements (the atom always has four free arms).

$$-\overset{\displaystyle |}{\underset{\displaystyle |}{C}}-$$

- Hydrogen (white ball) has only one electron, which needs two to fill the first shell in the electron cloud to become stable. Therefore, it needs one other electron. It can only join one other element (the atom always has one free arm).

H —

- Oxygen (red ball) has eight electrons, so it needs two more to complete the third electron shell; therefore, it can join two other elements (the atom always has two free arms).

—o—

Nature likes a balance, so in any atom, the number of protons and electrons must be equal to ensure there is no electrical charge.

If there are not enough electrons, the atom must seek electrons, attracting them by the charge. The atom does this by sharing electrons with another atom. When atoms share their electrons, a bond is formed. Chemical bonds can be of two different types. They are Ionic and Covalent bonds. Ionic compounds donate an electron and get a – or + charge, and a covalent bond share electron.

- **Ionic (electrovalent)** - The transfer (donate) of electrons from one atom to another forms these bonds. This transfer causes the formation of ions, which are electrically charged matter. *An example would be if person 'A' had $20.00, and person 'B' had $10.00, and both needed $15.00. Person 'A' would give a person 'B' $5.00, so both would have the correct amount.*

- **Covalent - The sharing of electrons, rather than the transfer of electrons from these bonds.** These bonds are called single, double, or triple, depending on the number of electrons shared.

An example would be if person 'A' had $10.00, and person 'B' had $10.00, and both needed $15.00. Both would have to share their money to have the correct amount.

Single Covalent Bond

- Stronger bond, saturated and sturdy.

E.g. Hydrogen

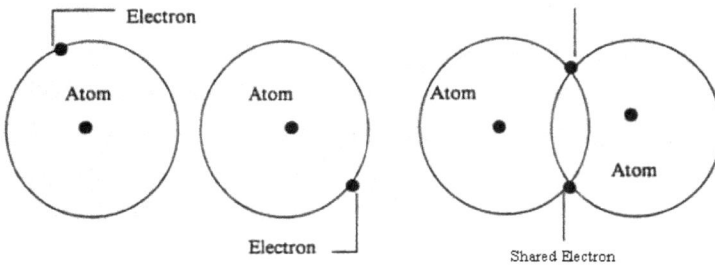

Hydrogen atom + Hydrogen atom = Hydrogen molecule H2
(Single covalent bond)

Double Covalent Bond

- More flexible, unsaturated, weaker bond.

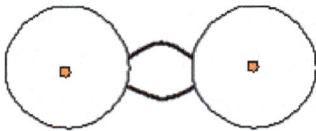

O - O
Oxygen Molecule O₂

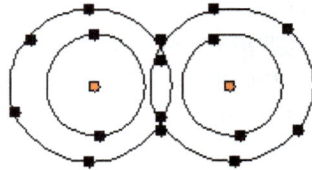

Double Covalent Bond

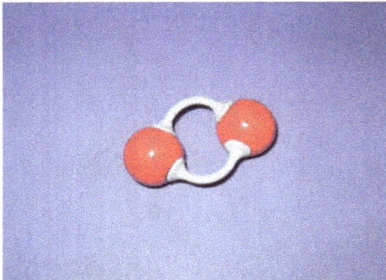

The oxygen atom (<u>element</u>) has 10 electrons.

An oxygen <u>molecule</u> has 16 electrons (the inner shell has two electrons.

Each outer shell has equivalent to eight electrons in each creating a double covalent bond).

H- *(single bond)*
O= *(double bond)*
C≡ *(triple bond)*

Molecular Compounds

Water H2O

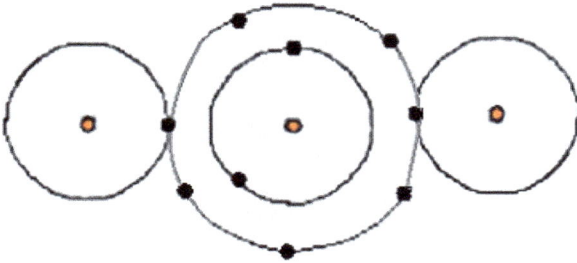

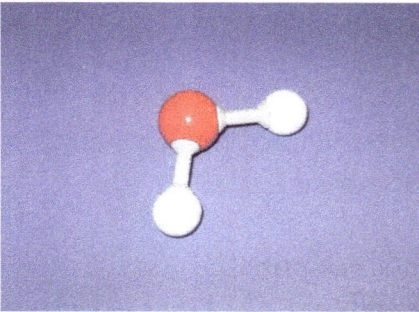

1 Oxygen element and 2 Hydrogen elements -sharing (two covalent bonds)

Biochemistry

Organic Chemistry

Definition: The chemistry of compounds that contain carbon (C).

All chemical compounds fall into one of two categories: **Organic** and **Inorganic.**

Organic chemistry has 133 compounds that contain Carbon (C). If it is not carbon-based, it is not alive.

A great variety of compounds are possible when considering that carbon compounds can bond with one or more of the following atoms: hydrogen (H) and oxygen (O).

Carbon is attracted to other carbon atoms and wants to bond. The more it bonds with other elements, the bigger and heavier the molecule.

The carbon atom bonds with other carbon atoms to form carbon chains and rings and join with hydrogen, oxygen, nitrogen, and sulfur atoms.

*The basic chemical elements in all living tissues are carbon (C), hydrogen (H), oxygen (0), and nitrogen (N)

Organic compounds are further divided into two types: **Aliphatic compounds** and **Aromatic compounds**. These are essential oils' two basic chemical building blocks or molecular formations. These are the molecules on which atoms are added to make more complex structures (creating the specifics of each essential oil).

The building blocks are:

ALIPHATIC / ACYCLIC

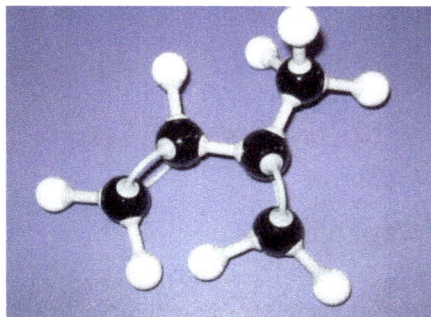

(Chain Building Blocks -open chain, no rings) or the "Isoprene Unit, " also known as the linear, means that in the molecule of organic chemical compounds, the carbon atoms form open chains that act as a base on which other atoms build to form more complex molecules. Simply put, the molecules form long chains like scaffolds on which other atoms can be added to to build different compounds.

> ➤ As it is linear, it does not have the stability of the aromatic compound.
> ➤ These chains or units combine to form progressively heavier and more volatile chemicals.
> ➤ The molecules contained in essential oils are 10 carbon atoms (with 2 isoprene units), 15 carbon atoms (with 3 isoprene units), or 20 carbon atoms (with 4 isoprene units) long.
> ➤ It forms the basic unit of all terpenes.
> ➤ It is always 5 carbon atoms linear or branched chain long.

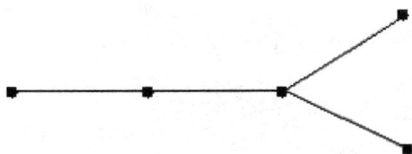

These molecules form the terpene class chemicals, including monoterpenes, sesquiterpenes, and diterpenes, which comprise the bulk of essential oils' constituents.

THE CYCLIC, AROMATIC, OR BENZENIC RING

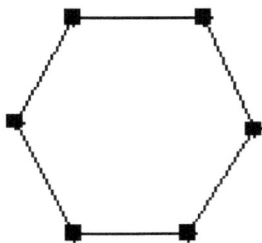

building block type (because the element formed is called benzene) or Phenol Rings (because phenols are formed from this base). This stable molecule forms the basis for several other chemotypes, including phenols, aldehydes, ketones, and organic acids.

These usually give off a noticeable odor or aroma. This means that the carbon atoms form a closed chain in the shape of a geometric figure,

➢ for example, a square, pentagon, or hexagon, the most characteristic aromatic molecule in essential oils is the characteristic hexagon of the benzene ring, to which a further chain of 4 carbons is attached to form the 10 carbon compounds present in essential oil constituents such as the phenols.

You can see the ring inside of the molecule that creates the 'Origanum.'

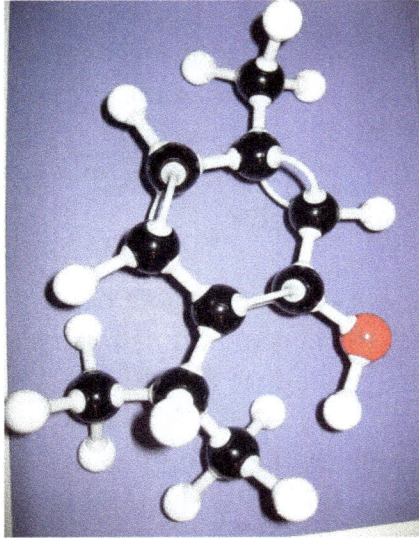

Written Formula of a Bond

Remember the three atoms that make up essential oils, C –carbon (4), H- hydrogen (1) & O- oxygen (2). These elements, when combined, are always written in this order alphabetically. Essential oil compounds are created by the essential oil molecules connecting the arms of the three atoms in combination with CH or CHO.

E.g., written formula of compounds

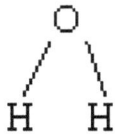

Water H2O   Carbon Dioxide CO2

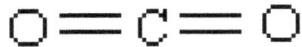

Isoprene always has five carbons, and in the end is always Hydrogen, no matter which way it is written.

C5 H8

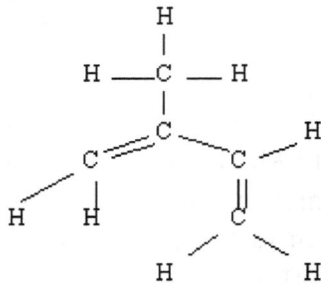

At the end of the carbon is a hydrogen

C5 H8

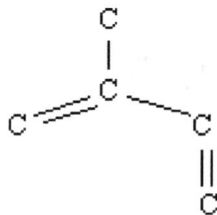

At the end of the carbon is a hydrogen

C5 H8

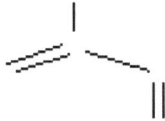

At the end of the carbon is a hydrogen

- ➢ R = the bond of carbon and hydrogen (one or more isoprene)
- ➢ R1 or R2 is when an isoprene is on either side of the other elements
- ➢ Carbon is always written first, then hydrogen, and last oxygen $C_{10}H_{16}O$

The combining of carbon molecules forms bonds in different ways. These are:

Alkanes (ane)-

These are a series of compounds that only contain single bonds between the carbon atoms in a straight chain structure. Molecules with all single bonds are saturated. They can rotate or spin constantly. These are <u>not</u> found in essential oils.

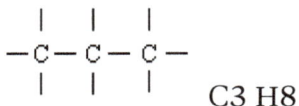

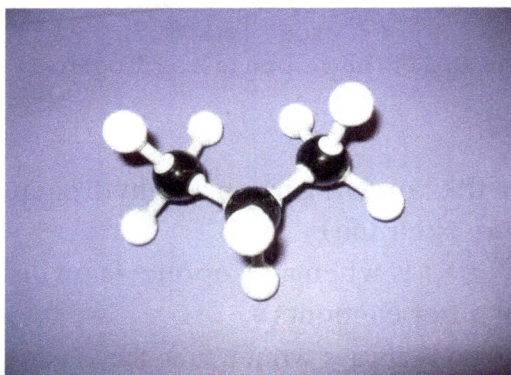

$$-\overset{\displaystyle |}{\underset{\displaystyle |}{C}}-\overset{\displaystyle |}{\underset{\displaystyle |}{C}}-\overset{\displaystyle |}{\underset{\displaystyle |}{C}}-$$

C3 H8

Alkenes (ene)- These are a series of compounds that contain double bonds between the carbon atoms in a straight chain structure. These molecules are said to be unsaturated as it has all double bonds. It does not have the capability of rotation.

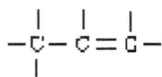

$$-\overset{|}{\underset{|}{C}} - \overset{|}{C} = \overset{|}{C} -$$

C3 H6

methane, ethane, propane

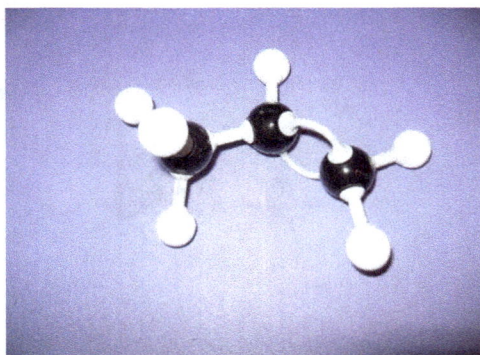

Alkynes (yne)- These are a series of compounds that contain triple bonds between the carbon atoms in a straight chain structure. This type of molecule is said to be unsaturated as they have triple bonds.

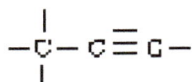

$$-\overset{|}{\underset{|}{C}}- C \equiv C -$$

C3 H4

ethene, propene, chloroethene

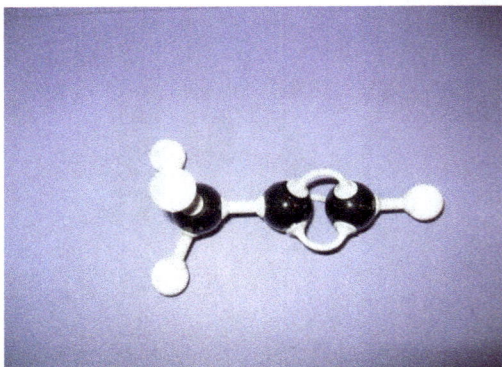

Cycloalkanes- These are alkanes that form a cyclic compound (ring) instead of straight chain compounds are saturated compounds. That is, they contain all single bonds between the carbon atoms. An example would be cyclopropane or C3H6.

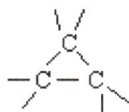

C3 H6

1,3-hexadien 5-yne

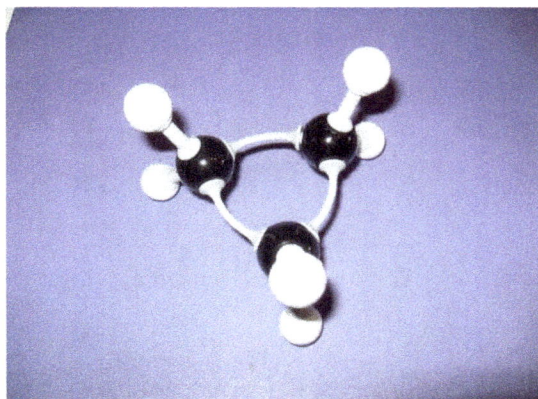

Cycloalkanes (circle – double bond) and Cycloalkynes (circle – triple bond)

Constituent	**Written Formula**

R=Isoprene   +

Acid $R - C \underset{OH}{\overset{O}{\diagup}}$

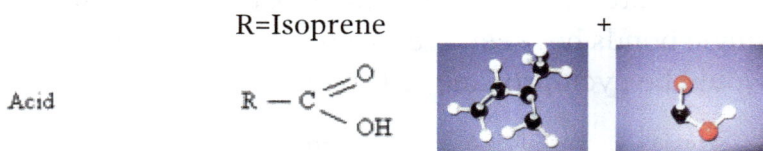

Alcohols $R - OH$

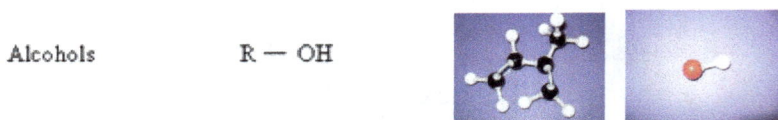

Aldehyde -Aliphatic $R - C \underset{H}{\overset{O}{\diagup}}$

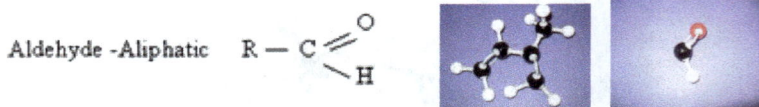

Ar =Aromatic (Benzenic) Ring +

Aldehyde -Aromatic $Ar - C \underset{H}{\overset{O}{\diagup}}$

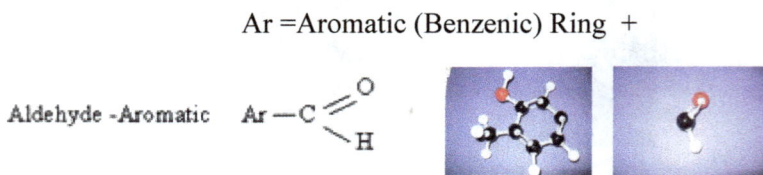

Esters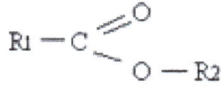

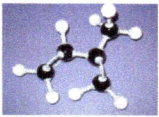 + 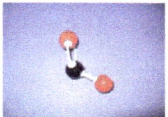 +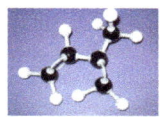

Ketone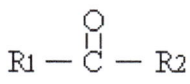

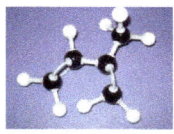 + 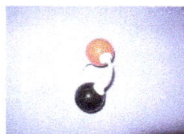 +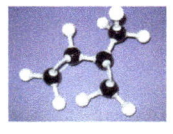

Oxide
1.8-Cineole

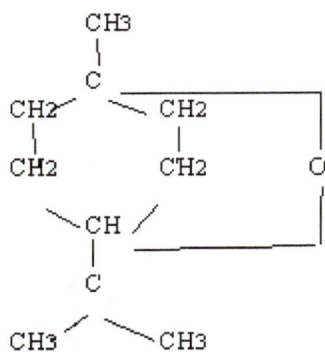

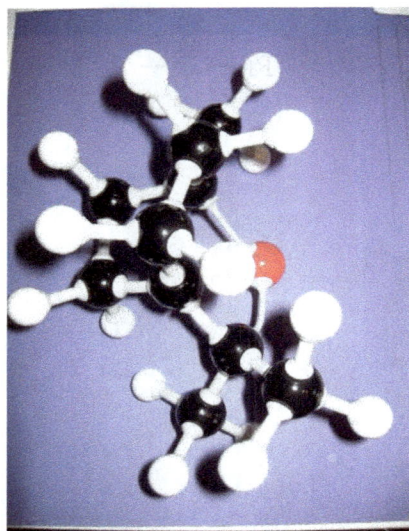

Phenol   Ar — OH

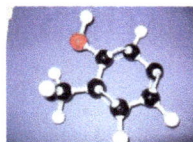

+

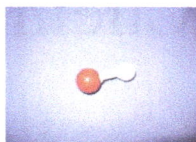

Terpene   They have 10, 15 or 20
(Hydrocarbons)   carbons rings or chains

Functional Groups/ Chemical Families

Functional groups are groups of atoms in a molecule, organic or inorganic, which are the ones most likely to undergo chemical change or a reaction.

It is the part that determines the chemical behavior of the molecule.

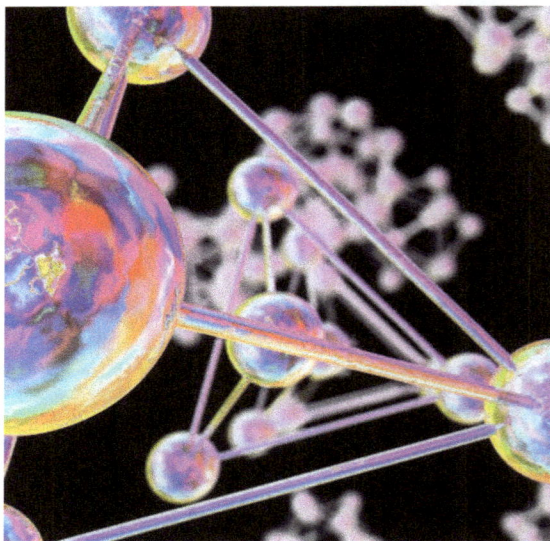

As we are constantly referring to the various chemicals that impact the effect of the essential oil, the terms functional group, chemotype, and constituent are interchangeable.

ORGANIC CHEMICAL FUNCTIONAL GROUPS (CONSTITUENTS)

Alcohol, Aldehyde, Amine, Amide, Carboxylic Acids, Ethers, Esters, Hydrocarbons (Alkanes, Alkenes, Alkynes), and Ketone.

Chemical Class	Common word endings
Acid	ic
Alcohols	ol or eol
Aldehyde	al
Esters	yl, il or ate
Ketone	one
Oxide	no ending
Phenol	ol
Terpene (hydrocarbons)	ene

The most common chemical constituents of essential oils fall into three main categories. They are:

1) **Hydrocarbons**

These are the terpenes. They contain just hydrogen atoms and carbon atoms.

These include:
- ➤ Monoterpenes
- ➤ Sesquiterpenes
- ➤ Diterpenes

2) Oxygenated Constituents.
They contain hydrogen atoms, carbon atoms, and oxygen atoms.
These include:
- ➤ aldehydes; aliphatic and aromatic
- ➤ ketones
- ➤ alcohols; monoterpenols and sesquiterpenols
- ➤ phenols
- ➤ oxides
- ➤ esters

3) Others are the
- ➤ acids; aliphatic and aromatic
- ➤ lactones (including coumarins & furocoumarins)
- ➤ phenylpropanes
- ➤ sulfur
- ➤ nitrogen

List of Essential Oils in each Family...

Following is a list of essential oils with each individual chemical that has a great percentage of that specific chemical and property.

Hydrocarbons

This group of chemicals (constituents) is made by adding hydrogen to aliphatic or isoprene units. It is composed of terpenes.

TERPENES

Terpenes are an important family of unsaturated naturally occurring aliphatic compounds based on the isoprene molecule. They commonly have up to 15 carbon atoms in the molecule.

Terpenes attract specific functional atomic groups and form other varied chemotypes. The terpene molecule is the basis for aldehydes, alcohols, ketones, and organic acids.

Some terpenes have a pleasant aroma and may be therapeutic. Their aroma ranges from a citrus fresh green note (all citrus oils, except Bergamot, contain high levels of terpenes) to an herbaceous, woody odor. They may be analgesic, hypotensive, and hormone-balancing properties.

A particularly important aspect of terpenes is that they may have a quenching effect on other molecules.

They may reduce the hazardous effects of other molecules. Never use a terpeneless oil. While it may have removed an irritant, it will also unbalance the oil!

Monoterpenes

Monoterpenes (ene)- or terpenes are molecules made up of two Isoprenes or 10 carbon atoms.

- ➤ **Alpha-pinene** (irritant-can cause skin eruption, delirium, and kidney damage) in balsam fir, carrot, cypress, juniper, saint john's wort, silver fir, tea tree, spearmint, and yarrow
- ➤ **Alpha-terpinene** (repels insects) in coriander, frankincense, lemon, oregano, scotch pine, St. John's wort, and sweet marjoram
- ➤ **Alpha sabinene and Gamma-terpinene** anti-viral
- ➤ **Beta-pinene** (repels insects) in carrot, myrtles, pennyroyal, savory, and scotch pine
- ➤ **Beta-phellandrene** (expectorant) in elemi and juniper
- ➤ **Camphene** (repels insects) in Ceylon citronella, Douglas fir, lemongrass, nutmeg, and Siberian fir
- ➤ **Delta-carene** (skin irritant, wide occurrence) in Douglas fir, Scotch pine, and Winter savory

- **Dipentene** (bactericide, skin irritant, and sensitizes, expectorant and sedative) in bergamot, lemongrass, palmarosa, and pine citronella
- **Limonene** Cancer prevention and treatment-d-limonene or perillyl (anticancer, antiseptic, anti-viral, bactericide, expectorant, fungicide, insecticide, irritant, sedative, and perfumery) in many oils, black pepper, carrot, caraway, and citrus peel
- **Myrcene** (bactericide, insecticide, and spasmolytic) in black pepper, cumin, fennel, frankincense, rose, scotch pine, and spearmint.
- **Para-cymene** muscle aches (analgesic, anti-flu, anti-rheumatic, diuretic, toxic to mammals, used externally for analgesic) in basil thymol, frankincense, lemon, thyme, and sweet marjoram
- **Pinene** increases energy level (antiseptic, bactericide, expectorant, fungicide, herbicide, and perfumery) in black pepper
- **Phellandrene** (irritant, ingestion causes vomiting and diarrhea) in eucalyptus, frankincense, ginger, spearmint, and summer savory
- **Sabinene** pain relief (analgesic, anti-arthritic, and anti-inflammatory) in cardamom,

cedarwood, geranium, ginger, juniper, laural, rose, scotch pine, thuja, and yarrow
➢ **Terpinolene** (perfumery and food additive, flammable) in clary sage, coriander, Douglas fir, elemi, green myrtle, orange, sweet marjoram, rosemary, verbonene, and winter savory
➢ **Y-terpinene** (anti-fungal) in coriander, cumin, lemon, oregano, sweet marjoram, and thyme

Therapeutic Properties:
- anti-viral,
- antiseptic in the air,
- bactericidal,
- expectorant (mucus),
- decongestant,
- pain relief,
- skin hygiene,
- stimulating,
- slightly analgesic,
- and good for the liver and gallbladder,
- Cancer prevention and treatment.

Contraindication:
- Possible skin irritants, especially mucous surfaces.

ESSENTIAL OILS HIGH IN MONOTERPENES

- Bergamot *(citrus bergamia)* and all citrus oils
- Black pepper *(piper nigrum)*
- Cypress *(cupressus sempervirens)*
- Many conifers (Balsam & Siberian Firs, Scotch Pine, White Pine, White Spruce, Black Spruce)
- Juniper Berry *(juniperus communis)*
- Tea Tree *(melaleuca alternifolia)*

Sesquiterpenes

Sesquiterpenes (ene) – are molecules made of three Isoprenes or 15 carbon atoms.

They contribute to the lasting odor of the essential oil or the base note, as most sesquiterpenes consist of large, slowly evaporating molecules.

> ➢ **Alpha-bisabolol** cellular re-growth, liver stimulant
> ➢ **Aromadendrene** (some anti-fungal, cancer preventative) in E. gobules, tea tree, sage, and winter savory.
> ➢ **Beta-caryophyllene** (anti-inflammatory, insectifuge, perfumern, spasmoltic) in black pepper, cajeput, cedarwood, cinnamon, clove, eucalyptus, hyssop, lavender, lemon, litsea, marjoram, melissa, niaouli, pennyroyal, tea tree, and verbena
> ➢ **Bisabolene** (perfumern) in lemon, lime, carrot, and sandalwood
> ➢ **Cadinene** (perfumery/scent) in cedarwood, myrrh, myrtle, niaouli, patchouli, tea tree, and spruce
> ➢ **Cedrene** (cancer preventative and perfumery) in atlas cedar, cypress, and Texas cedarwood

- ➢ **Cedrol** vein tonic
- ➢ **Carotol** glandular stimulant, immunostimulant
- ➢ **Chamazulene** (anti-inflammatory, antispasmodic, stimulates granulation tissue formation in wound healing) in chamomile and yarrow.
- ➢ **Farnesene** (anti-inflammatory and insectifuge) in linden blossom and ylang ylang
- ➢ **Farensol** anti-cancer
- ➢ **Germacrene** (pheromonal) in ginger, lemon, melissa, pennyroyal, pine, yarrow, ylang-ylang, and verbena
- ➢ **Humulene** (anti-inflammatory, insectifuge, perfumery, and spamolytic) in black pepper, clove, laural, melissa, myrtle, and patchouli
- ➢ **Nerolidol** colon tumors
- ➢ **Spatulenol** fungicide
- ➢ **Viridiflorol** estrogen like, vein tonic

Therapeutic Properties:
- slightly anti-cancer,
- analgesic,
- antiseptic,
- anti-allergic,
- anti-phlogistic,
- bactericidal,
- hypotensive,
- liver stimulating,

- calming,
- anti-inflammatory,
- antiviral,
- anti-allergenic,
- antispasmodic,
- balancing,
- relaxes cramps,
- neuronal,
- slightly lowers blood pressure,
- vascular,
- astringent,
- and anti-fungal.

Contraindications:

- Black Pepper, if have a kidney issue

ESSENTIAL OILS HIGH IN SESQUITERPENES

- Balsam Copaiba (copaifera officinalis)
- Ginger (zingiber officinale)
- Cedarwood (juniperus virginiana)
- Manuka (leptospermum scoparium ct east cape)
- Melissa (melissa officinalis)
- Vetiver (vetiveria zizanoides)
- Myrrh (commiphora myrrha)
- Patchouli (pogostemon cablin)
- Rhododendron (rhododendron anthopogon)

- Ylang Ylang (Complete) (cananga odorata var genuina)
- Black Pepper (piper nigrum)

Diterpenes

Diterpenes (ene)- These constituents are rare in essential oils because the size of the molecule interferes with distillation. These constituents can be found in Camphor and Clary Sage essential oils.

Diterpenes - are molecules made up of four Isoprenes or 20 carbon atoms.

Therapeutic Properties:
- slightly bactericidal
- and expectorant.

Contra-indications:
- Terpenes may be irritating to the skin.
- A special note - Dextrolimonenes are thought to be quenchers.

ESSENTIAL OILS HIGH IN MONOTERPENOLS

- Camphor *(Cinnamomum camphora)*
- Clary Sage *(Salvia sclarea)*

Alcohols

= OXYGEN + ALIPHATICS

The addition of a hydroxyl group, -OH, to terpenes results in an alcohol, which is identified with the name ending in "ol." *These oils are good to use on the elderly and children.* Three types of alcohol can be formed depending on the terpene and hydroxyl group it bonds to. If you add -OH to an aliphatic chain, you get:

Monoterpenols

Monoterpenols- results from monoterpenes. These alcohols include terpineol 4, geraniol, linalool, and menthol.

- ➢ **Borneo**l (analgesic, anti-inflammatory, bactericidal, expectorant, and toxic to mammals) in lavender, lemongrass, and rosemary.
- ➢ **Citronellol** (antiseptic, bactericide, fungicide, perfumery, and sedative) in E. citriodora, geranium, ginger, and rose.

> **Geraniol** (antiseptic, cancer-preventative, embryotoxic, fungicide, insectifuge, perfumery (rose scent), sedative) in carrot seed, cinnamon, geranium, lemongrass, neroli, palmarosa, petitgrain, and rose.
> **Linalol** sedating, relaxant (antiseptic, bactericide, cancer-preventative, fungicide, insectifuge, perfumery, sedative, and spasmoltic, vaso-constictive, anesthetic) in basil, carrot seed, clary sage, coriander, geranium, ginger, jasmine, lavendin, spike lavender, lavender, lime, marjoram, neroli, palmarosa, petitgrain, and rosewood.
> **Menthol** (analgesic, anesthetic, anti-inflammatory, anti-neuralgic, anti-rheumatic, antiseptic, carminative, CNS-depressant, decongestant, perfumery, and spasmolytic, vasoconstrictive, anesthetic) in camphor, pennyroyal, peppermint, and spearmint.
> **Terpinene-4-ol** (relaxant, antiseptic, bacteriostatic, fungicide, herbicide, and insecticide) in juniper, lavender, marjoram, nutmeg, and ravensara.
> **Terpinene and alpha-terpeneol** (vasoconstrictive, anesthetic, antiseptic, bactericide, expectorant, insectifuge, and perfumery) in basil, chamomile R, clary sage,

cypress, lavender, lime, marjoram, niaoulí, petitgrain, pine, and ravensara.

Therapeutic Properties:
- antibacterial,
- antiseptic,
- diuretic,
- immunostimulant,
- uplifting,
- anti-infectious,
- anti-viral,
- antifungal,
- anti-infective,
- anti-spasmodic,
- immune system balancer,
- stimulating (CNS),
- tonic for the liver and nerves,
- warming,
- and a good general tonic.

Contraindications:
- The alcohol is nonirritating to the skin and appears to have no contra-indications at low dilutions.
- They are good to use on children.

ESSENTIAL OILS HIGH IN MONOTERPENOLS

- Peppermint *(mentha x piperita)*
- Lavender *(lavandula angustifolia)*
- Clary sage *(salvia sclarea)*
- Geranium rose *(Rosa x damascena/pelargonium x asperum)*
- Neroli *(Citrus aurantium var. amara)*
- Palmarosa *(cymbopogon martinii var. motia)*
- Rose absolute *(rosa x damascena)*
- Spike lavender *(lavandula latifolia)*
- Sweet marjoram *(origanum majorana)*
- Tea tree *(melaleuca alternifolia)*
- Fragonia *(agonis fragrans)*
- Petitgrain *(citrus aurantium var. amara or bigaradia)*

Sesquiterpenols

Sesquiterpenols - from sesquiterpenes. These alcohols are decongestants to the circulatory system and a tonic. Some have specific qualities that relate to specific functions, such as stimulating the heart.

➢ **Bisabolol and alpha-bisabolol** (analgesic, anti-inflammatory, reduces histamine reaction (hay fever and asthma), spasmolytic) in chamomile G
➢ **Farnesol** (perfumery) in citronella, jasmine, lemongrass, linden blossom, neroli, palmarosa, rose, and ylang ylang
➢ **Santalol** (perfumery and urinary antiseptic) in sandalwood

Therapeutic Properties:
- anti-inflammatory,
- hormone balancing,
- hypotensive,
- immunostimulants,
- tonics to the CNS and skin.

Contraindications:
- non-irritating to the skin and appear to have no contra-indications at low dilutions.

ESSENTIAL OILS HIGH IN SESQUITERPENOLS

- Carrot seed *(daucus carota)*
- Cedarwood *(juniperus virginiana)*
- German chamomile *(matricaria recutita)*
- Ginger *(zingiber officinale)*
- Patchouli *(pogostemon cablin)*
- Sandalwood *(santalum album)*
- Vetiver *(vetiveria zizanoides)*

Diterpenols

Diterpenols - from diterpenes. These are heavy molecules, and few are found in essential oils because they do not readily evaporate in the distillation process.

Therapeutic Properties:
- They are like human steroids and appear to balance the hormone system. An example of this group is Sciareol, which is found in clary sage.

Alcohols are also classified as terpinols (C-b), sesquiterpenols (C-is), and diterpinols (C-20).

ESSENTIAL OILS HIGH IN DITERPENOLS

- Clary Sage *(Salvia sclarea)*

Phenols

Oxygen and Either Aliphatic (chain) or Aromatic (ring) Alcohols

= Oxygen and Aromatic (Benzene Rings)

Dilute!

Phenols are formed when the hydroxyl group joins a carbon atom in a benzene or aromatic ring.

Phenols are responsible for the fragrance of many oils, and they extend their range. Phenols are stronger and more active than alcohol. Unfortunately, they also end with an "ol" (or "ole" in a phenolic ether). Some phenols include carvacrol, eugenol, and thymol.

> **Carvacrol** (antiseptic, antifungal, anti-inflammatory, bactericide, carminative, expectorant, spasmolytic) in oregano and savory
> **Methyl Eugenol** (anesthetic, anticonvulsant, antidote (strychinine), antifeedant, antiseptic, bactericide, cancer-preventative, carcinogenic, fungistatic, fungicide, insectifuge, myorelaxant, narcotic and sedative) in citronella, snakeroot,

bay leaf, cassis, tea tree, hyacinth, bay allspice, and exotic basil.

➤ **Thymol** (anesthetic, anti-bronchitic, anti-inflammatory, anti-rhematic, anti-septic, bactericide, carminative, deodorant, expectorant, fungicide, spasmolytic, urinary antiseptic) in camphor, origanum, and red/white thyme.

Therapeutic Properties:
- very strong antiseptics,
- antivirals,
- antifungals,
- analgesic,
- anti-inflammatory,
- anti-infective,
- anti-septic,
- antispasmodics,
- anti-hematoma,
- anti-hemorrhoidal,
- bactericidal (best),
- cholesterol-lowering,
- citatrisants,
- expectorants,
- immunostimulants,
- parasiticides,
- hormone-like,
- mucolytic,

- raise temperature,
- hypertensive,
- wound healing,
- and sedatives.

Contraindications:
- They do pose a risk of skin irritation
- and can, in large dosages, damage the liver.

ESSENTIAL OILS HIGH IN PHENOLS

- Clove bud *(eugenia caryophyllata)*
- Oregano *(origanum vulgare)*
- Cinnamon leaf *(cinnamomum zeylanicum)*
- Holy Basil *(ocimum sanctum ct eugenol)*

Aldehydes

Aliphatic Structure + Carbonyl Group + Hydrogen Atom = Aldehyde

Aromatic Ring + Carbonyl Group + Hydrogen Atom = Aldehyde

Aldehydes are formed from both the aliphatic chain and aromatic rings. Aldehydes are formed by adding a carbonyl group (=O) and a hydrogen (-H) atom to the same carbon atom in the aliphatic chain or the aromatic ring. They often have a powerful odor. They are easily identified by the "al" ending of their name, such as citral, or in the case of aromatic aldehydes, the word aldehyde, such as in cinnamic aldehyde found in the oil of cinnamon.

Terpenic aldehydes are very aromatic and are used by the perfume industry extensively.

- ➤ **Anisaldehyde** (insecticide and fungicide) in fennel and mimosa
- ➤ **Cinnamaldehyd** (antiulcer, cancer-preventative, CNS depressant, CNS stimulant, hypotensive, insectice, perfumery, sedative, and spasmolytic)

in cinnamon bark, lavender, myrrh, and
patchouli

➢ **Citronellal** (antiseptic, bactericidal,
embryotoxic, insectifuge, perfumery, and
sedative) in citronella, E. citriodora, E. radiate,
grapefruit, geranium, lemon, lemongrass,
melissa, rose.

➢ **Citral** (calming to the CNS, anti-histaminic,
antiseptic, bactericide, cancer-preventative,
fungicide, herbicide, perfumery, sedative, and
synthesis of vitamin A) in citronellal, E. radiate,
java citronella, lemon, lemongrass, lime,
marjoram, melissa, palmarosa, scotch pine, and
verbena.

➢ **Cuminaldehyde** (bactericide, fungicide, and
perfumery) in cinnamon bark, cumin, and
myrrh

➢ **Geranial** (antiseptic, bactericidal, flavor, and
perfumery) in E radiate, ginger, lemon,
lemongrass, lemon verbena, palmarosa,
petitgrain, and orange

➢ **Neral** (antiseptic, bactericide, and perfumery) in
lemon, lemongrass, orange, and verbena

➢ **Trans-2-hexenal** anti-cancerous (melanoma)

Therapeutic Properties:
- anti-inflammatory,
- anti-infectious,
- anti-bacterial,
- antiviral,
- anti-septic,
- anti-fungal,
- calming on the CNS,
- hypotensive,
- relaxants,
- vasodilators,
- and stimulants for the endocrine system. The citral molecule of the aldehyde group has an antiseptic action.
- Aldehydes, in general, have a sedative effect on the nervous system
- and generally, temperature reduction.
- Aromatic Aldehydes stimulate on the CNS, digestive system, sexual organs, and muscles.

Contraindications:
- may be a skin irritant or skin sensitizer.
- experience has shown that aldehydes may irritate the skin when isolated, but not when used as part of oil.
- The other constituents, terpenes, appear to quench the negative effects.

It should be noted that if the essential oil were not stored correctly, the aldehydes would become useless acids and remove their therapeutic properties.

ESSENTIAL OILS HIGH IN ALDEHYDES

- Lemongrass (cymbopogon flexuosus)
- Melissa *(melissa officinalis)*
- Citronella *(cymbopogon winterianus)*

Ketones

Aliphatic structure + Carbonyl Group = Ketones
Aromatic Ring + Carbonyl Group = Ketones

Ketones in high amounts can be potentially neurotoxic. Most dangerous essential oils are high in Ketones.

Dilute!

Ketones are created when a carbonyl group (=0) attaches to a carbon atom of either an aliphatic chain or aromatic ring. Ketones can vary in odor from celery-like to violet-like.

Ketones are another functional group commonly referred to as a toxic constituent. *Generally, they are considered dangerous by some authors.* However, not all ketones are dangerous. Ketones are found in plants and recognized for their benefits in relieving respiratory complaints (such as hyssop). Other ketones include camphone, carvone, menthone, methyl heptanone, and pinocamphone.

> ➢ **Camphor** (analgesic, mild anesthetic, antiseptic, cancer-preventative, carminative, CNS –

stimulant, convulsant, expectorant, herbicide, insectifuge, stimulant, irritant, toxic to humans) in clary sage, juniper, marjoram, lavendin, lavender, lavender spike, laural, oregano, rosemary, sage, savory, thyme, and yarrow.

➢ **Carvone** (antiseptic, cancer-preventative, carminative, CNS-stimulant, insecticice, insectifuge) in caraway, coriander, elemi, spearmint, and tagerts

➢ **Menthone** (analgesic, antiseptic, cancer–preventative, sedative) in geranium, pennyroyal, peppermint, and spearmint

➢ **Pulegone** (anthistamic, anti-asthmatic, cancer-preventative, hepatatoxic, herbicide, insectifuge, insecticide, and sedative) in pennyroyal and peppermint

➢ **Thujone** (canvulsant, epileptogenic, hallucinogenic, herbicide, respiroinhibator, ingestion may cause convulsions) in blue tansey, tarragon, and yarrow

➢ **Verbenone** (caused by oxidation of alpha-pinene –old oils with pinene) in E globules, rosemary, verbena, and verbenone

Therapeutic Properties:
- break down mucus and fat
- and assist in the formation of scar tissue.
- Some may be

- o anti-hematoma,
- o abortifacient,
- o analgesic,
- o anticoagulant,
- o antifungal,
- o anti-inflammatory,
- o bactericidal,
- o cicatrisant,
- o digestive,
- o expectorant,
- o lipolytic,
- o mucolytic,
- o neurotoxic,
- o relaxant,
- o sedative,
- o stimulant,
- o and wound healing.

Contraindications:
- Ketones must be used with caution.
- Several are neurotoxic.
- Pinocamphone, found in hyssop, may provoke an epileptic seizure in people predisposed to them
- Several may encourage a miscarriage if too much is used. (Large amounts of this oil may have to be consumed for it to have a toxic neurologic effect.)

- High dosages of ketones stimulate the CNS.
- Prolonged use and buildup of ketones in the system can cause CNS depression.

To be safe, always use well-diluted, not more than 5 drops per 25 ml carrier oil.

It has never been recorded or documented that these oils have ever caused a toxic effect on a human being. That does not mean that they have not. Researchers discovered a toxic effect in laboratory testing on guinea pigs and rats.) An aromatherapist always errors on the side of safety and would not use any oil that may pose a threat.

Scientists do not believe that all ketones are dangerous and have shown that the four different types of structure found in ketones change the value of the oil and, likely, the hazards.

ESSENTIAL OILS HIGH IN KETONES

- Rosemary ct camphor *(Rosmarinus officinalis ct camphor)*
- Spike lavender *(Lavandula latifolia)*
- Peppermint *(Mentha x piperita)*
- Vetiver *(Vetiveria zizanoides)*
- Turmeric *(Curcuma longa)*

OTHER COMPOUNDS AND COMBINATIONS

Acids

Organic Acids + Alcohol = Esters + Water

Acids are also called carboxylic acids. They can be either organic or inorganic. Inorganic acids (sulphuric acid) are dangerous and are not found in essential oils.

Organic acids are and can be beneficial. They are found in oils but only in small amounts. They are usually located in a combined state with esters. They have an affinity with water, so they are usually found in hydrosols of essential oils that contain them.

- ➢ **Benzonic acid** (allergenic, antiseptic, bactericide, expectorant, fungicide, and insectifuge) in benzoin and vetiver
- ➢ **Cinnamic acid** (may cause contact dermatitis, anesthetic, bactericide, cancer-preventative, laxative, and spasmolytic) in benzoin and cinnamon
- ➢ **Palmitic acid** (antioxidant) in vetiver

Therapeutic Properties:
- anti-inflammatory,
- regenerate mucous membranes
- and stimulates the digestive and muscular systems.

Contraindications:
- They have no contra-indications except for methyl salicylate. They often provide the essential oil with a fruity aroma.

ESSENTIAL OILS HIGH IN ACIDS

- Benzoin (*Styrax benzoin*)
- Cinnamon (*Cinnamomum verum*)

Esters

Esters are found in most essential oils. They are formed by the interaction between organic acids and alcohol. Water is another by-product. Therefore, you only find esters in oils with acids. It is also possible for a reaction to occur between esters and water, resulting in acids and alcohol. Most likely, a constant change between states is always occurring.

- **Benzyl acetate** (emetic and laxative) in clove bud, jasmine, and ylang ylang
- **Bornyl acetate** (bactericide, expectorant, bronchial, insectifuge, and nasal inhalant) in cistus, coriander, fir, juniper, lavandin, pine, rosemary, sage, spikenard, and spruce
- **Geranyl acetate** (insect attraction and perfumery) in citronella, eucalyptus, geranium, lemongrass, palmarosa, petitgrain, and neroli
- **Isobutyl angelate** grand antispasmodic
- **Linalyl acetate** anti-viral (perfumery) in bergamot, clary sage, lavender, marjoram, neroli, petitgrain, and ylang ylang
- **Methyl salicylate** (allergenic, analgesic, anti-inflammatory, antirheumatic, cancer-preventative, carminative) in birch and wintergreen

➤ **Neryl actetate** (antiflu) in clary sage, helichrysum, lemon, neroli, and petitgrain

Therapeutic Properties:
- antispasmodic,
- sedative,
- antifungal,
- anti-inflammatory,
- balancing,
- cicatrisant,
- and immune-modulant.

Contraindications:
- The esters are generally safe to use, except for methyl salicylate, which is found in wintergreen and birch.

ESSENTIAL OILS HIGH IN ESTERS

- Wintergreen *(gaultheria fragrantissima)*
- Bergamot *(citrus bergamia)*
- Cardamom *(elettaria cardamomum)*
- Roman Chamomile *(chamaemelum nobile)*
- Clary Sage *(salvia sclarea)*
- Rose Geranium *(rosa x damascena/pelargonium x asperum)*
- Jasmine Absolute *(kasminum sambac)*

Ethers

Also called Phenol-methyl-ethers, ethers are rarely found in essential oils. They occur when an oxygen atom joins phenolic alcohol with methyl alcohol. The starting point is cinnamic acid. Depending on the hydrophilic quality, ethers are said to be hot or mild. The more hydrophilic, the hotter it is. Hot ones will cause skin irritation and liver and kidney toxicity. Mild ones may cause skin irritation and toxicity. (Note: some refer to these as phenylpropanes).

> ➤ hot - cinnamon, clove, and nutmeg
> ➤ mild - Basil, Jasmine, and Tarragon

Ethers are rarely found in oils, but when they are, their therapeutic values are they are analgesic, antispasmodic, anti-infective, anti-parasitic, balancing, calming, relaxing, sedative, stimulating, and soothing.

> ➤ **Anethol** (bactericide, carminative, expectorant, fungicide, and gastro-stimulant) in anise, coriander, fennel, and tarragon
> ➤ **Eugenol** (analgesic, anti-inflammatory, antiseptic in dentistry, CNS depressant, fungicide, sedative, spasmolytic, and skeletal muscle relaxant

> **Methyl chavicol** (anesthetic, anticonvulsant, hepatocarcinogenic, insecticide, perfumery, stimulate liver regeneration) in basil, fennel, tarragon

Therapeutic Properties:
- antiallergenic,
- antidepressant,
- anti-infectious,
- antispasmodic,
- balancing ANS,
- and immunomodulant.

Contraindications:
- liver

ESSENTIAL OILS HIGH IN ETHERS

- Sweet Fennel *(foeniculum vulgare)*

Oxides

= OXIDES
ALIPHATIC STRUCTURES + OXYGEN

Oxides are binary compounds formed between oxygen and other elements. In the case of essential oils, the oxygen binds with 2 carbon atoms. Some chemists argue that some oxides are phenols or phenol ethers. Oxides are difficult to distill. By far, the most important oxide is 1,8 cineol, which is known as eucalyptol and is found in eucalyptus and cinnamon. Another is methyl chavicol, found in basil. Oxides are rare in oils except for eucalyptol. Some oxides have "oxide" at the end of their name or end with an "ole," making identification easier. Unfortunately, not all do.

- ➤ **1,4-cineole** in tea tree
- ➤ **1,8-cineole** (anesthetic, antibronchitic, anticatarrh, anti-inflammatory, antiseptic, bactericide, CNS-stimulant, counterirritant, expectorant, fungicide, heptatonic, herbicide, hypotensive, insectifuge and sedative) in eucalyptus, ginger, lavedin, lavender, marjoram, niaouli, peppermint, ravensara, rosemary, sage, spearmint, spike lavender, tea tree, and thyme

> ➤ **caryophylene oxide** (anti-inflammatory) in black pepper, clary sage, clove, eucalyptus radiata, marjoram, myrtle, lavender,

Therapeutic Properties:
- expectorant,
- analgesic,
- antirheumatic,
- antifungal,
- antiviral,
- anti-spasmodic,
- anti-inflammatory,
- mucolytic,
- and expectorant making it useful for coughs, colds, and congestion,
- parasidic

Contraindications:
- the oxides can provoke excessive coughing
- and, in some cases, trap secretions in the bronchial tree.
- They can also irritate the skin (especially on young children), and if the content is 10% or higher, they should be used with care.

ESSENTIAL OILS HIGH IN OXIDES

- Cardamom *(elettaria cardamomum)*
- Eucalyptus Globulus *(eucalyptus globulus)*
- Fragonia *(agonis fragrans)*
- Spike Lavender *(lavandula latifolia)*
- Ravintsara *(cinnamomum camphora 1,8 cineole)*
- Rosalina *(melaleuca ericifolia)*

Lactones

Lactones are large and difficult to steam distill. They result from the addition of an oxide to a ketone molecule, and as a result, they are a variety of ketone. They are found most often in expressed essential oils or if produced by solvent.

They are not usually found in essential oils and are usually in minute quantities.

- ➢ **Bergaptene** (anti-inflammatory, antiseptic, fungicide, hypotensive, insecticide, phototoxic, and spasmolytic) in angelica seed, bergamot, coriander seed, fennel, grapefruit, lemon, lime, and sweet and bitter orange
- ➢ **Courmarins** (hemorrhagic effect, antifungal, anti-tumor, anti-inflammatory, immunostimulant, hypnotic, and sedative) in spikenard
- ➢ **Nepetalactone** sedation
- ➢ **Umbelliferone** (antifungal, antihistaminic, antiseptic, cancer-preventative, fungicide, and sunscreen) in angelica root, anise seed, coriander, dill, and fennel

Therapeutic Properties:
- antifungal,
- anti-infectious,
- antipyretic,
- anti-inflammatory,
- anthelmintic,
- highly mucolytic,
- hepatic (liver tonic),
- mucolytic,
- and release emotions.

Contraindications:
- allergies,
- they have limited contra-indications. They are generally considered nontoxic.
- In essential oils with large percentages of lactones, neurotoxicity, and skin irritations are of concern.
- They are also responsible for photosensitivity.

ESSENTIAL OILS HIGH IN LACTONES
- Yarrow *(Achillea millefolium)*

Coumarins

Coumarins are formed by the addition of lactone to a benzenic kernel. Coumarins have a special relationship with the CNS.

Therapeutic Properties:
- sedative and calming while uplifting and refreshing.
- anticoagulating,
- hypotensive,
- anti-lymphoemic,
- and reduce edema,
- anticonvulsive,
- anticoagulant,
- relaxant,
- Some are antiviral and antifungal.

Contraindications:
- can cause photosensitivity.

ESSENTIAL OILS HIGH IN COUMARINS
- Citrus essential oils.

Furocoumarins

Furocoumarins are a type of coumarins. A good example is bergaptene, found in bergamot oil.

Therapeutic Properties:
- sedative and calming while uplifting and refreshing.
- anticoagulating,
- hypotensive,
- anti-lymphoemic,
- and reduce edema,
- anticonvulsive,
- anticoagulant,
- relaxant,
- Some are antiviral and antifungal.

Contraindications:
- can cause photosensitivity.

ESSENTIAL OILS HIGH IN FUROCOUMARINS
- Bergamot (*Citrus bergamia)*

Chemical Overview

Acids	Deodorant
Alcohol	Antiviral, bactericidal, Tonifying, energizing
Aliphatic Aldehyde	Refreshing, antiseptic, antifungal
Aromatic Aldehyde	Warming, antiseptic, antifungal
Esters	Balancing, soothing for skin
Ether	Anti-spasmodic
Ketone	Cooling, decongestant, analgesic
Lactones & Coumarins	Balancing, decongestant, photosensitive
Oxide	Expectorant, respiratory decongestant, diuretic
Monoterpenes	Skin tonic, digestion, liver
Phenol	Stimulant, antiviral, aggressive
Sesquiterpene	Balancing, soothing, digestion, warming
Terpene	Drying, antiviral

Advanced Aromatherapy Procedure

1st Step:
You will need to know which is the main '**System**' of the body that the condition or disease is created. Look up the condition in the **Textbook: 'Prescription for Nutritional Healing'** or online and read what system of the body created the issue.

2nd Step:
Create a Therapeutic Cross-Referencing Sheet (TCRS - taught in the Magic of Aromatherapy book), and add two other systems (you can look at the essential oils listed under the system on page 55) or you can add any conditions that relate to the issue.

Therapeutic Cross Reference Form

CLIENTS NAME: _____   *Essential Oils Blend*

Visit # _____	Signature _____			Date: _____	
MAIN CONDITION			MAIN SYSTEM		SECOND SYSTEM
Stress					
Bas	Cha	Ben			
Ber	Ger	C/W			
C/S	Hys	Fra			
Lem	Jun	Imm			
Man	Lav	Jas			
Ora	Mar	L/B			
Pet	Mel	Myr			
Thy	Pep	Ner			
Y'ar	Pin	Pat			
	R/M	Ros			
	R/W	S/W			
		Vet			
		Y/Y			

Contra-Indications:

BLEND: Acute ___ Chronic ___ Synergistic ___   Cream ___ Lotion ___ Oil ___ Spritzer ___ Other _____

OIL -	OIL -	OIL -	OIL -	OIL -	Carrier Oil Used:	5% of the other Oil:
# of Drops ___	# of Drops ___	# of Drops ___	# of Drops ___	# of Drops ___	Crystals:	Herbs:

Practitioner

3rd Step:

Find the best essential oils for that system(s). Follow the procedure for TCRS.

4th Step:

Cross out any essential oils that could be contra-indicated.

5th Step:

From the TCRS, compare the chemical constituent percentages. Choose the best essential oil(s) suited to the person's issue or condition based on the percentage of active constituents.

Chemical	Properties
Acids	Deodorant
Alcohol	Antiviral, bactericidal, Tonifying, energizing
Aliphatic Aldehyde	Refreshing, antiseptic, antifungal
Aromatic Aldehyde	Warming, antiseptic, antifungal
Esters	Balancing, soothing for skin
Ether	Anti-spasmodic
Ketone	Cooling, decongestant, analgesic
Lactones & coumarins	Balancing, decongestant, photosensitive
Oxide	Expectorant, respiratory decongestant, diuretic
Monoterpenes	Skin tonic, digestion, liver
Phenol	Stimulant, antiviral, aggressive
Sesquiterpene	Balancing, soothing, digestion, warming
Terpene	Drying, anti-viral

To see a full chart of Essential Oil Chemical Constituent Percentages, go to my website page:

https://constancesantego.ca/education/secrets-from-a-healer-series/magic-of-aromatherapy/constituents-properties/

6th Step:
Create your blend.
Use the same recipes you were taught in the "Magic of Aromatherapy" book for creating the blend.

Miscellaneous

Grid System

Piere Franchomme, a French chemist and researcher, spent years determining or mapping plant chemical constituents. He attributed many, if not all, a plant's therapeutic properties to the polarity of the essential oil constituents. He, with others, Roger Jollois, Daniel Penoel, and J. Mars, developed a grid system that clearly demonstrated the strength of polarity and its solubility. By studying these grids, an aromatherapist can blend to strengthen or weaken certain properties.

Rosemary Caddy has developed a system and grid pattern like the above-mentioned, which includes color.

There are some that believe this belief system is only a hypothesis.

> ➢ The horizontal axis represents the solubility of the constituent. The far left represents those that repel water (insoluble). They are called

hydrophobic or lipophilic. The far right tends to attract water and is called hydrophilic. As all essential oils are soluble to some degree, there is no location that is totally not soluble.

➤ The vertical axis represents the polarity of components.

➤ The center is neutral.

➤ Those at the bottom have a strong tendency to take on electrons and are called electrophilic (negative). These oils tend to be stimulating.

➤ Those at the top have a strong tendency to release or give up electrons (positive) and are called nucleophilic. These oils tend to be calming.

➤ Positive and negative charged elements are attracted to each other.

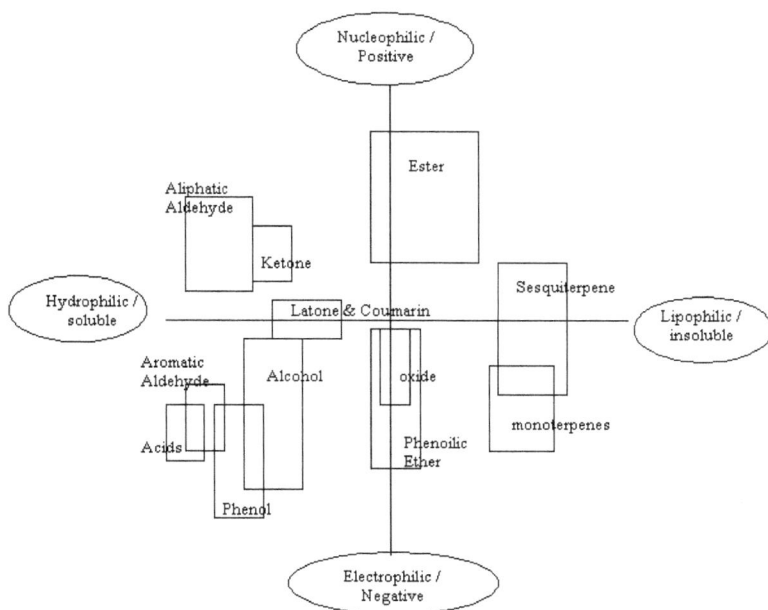

About Rosemary Caddy

One of the quickest ways to create a blend using Chemical Constituent Percentages is by purchasing Rosemary Caddy's software, https://www.ccprofiles.co.uk/essential-oils-software.htm

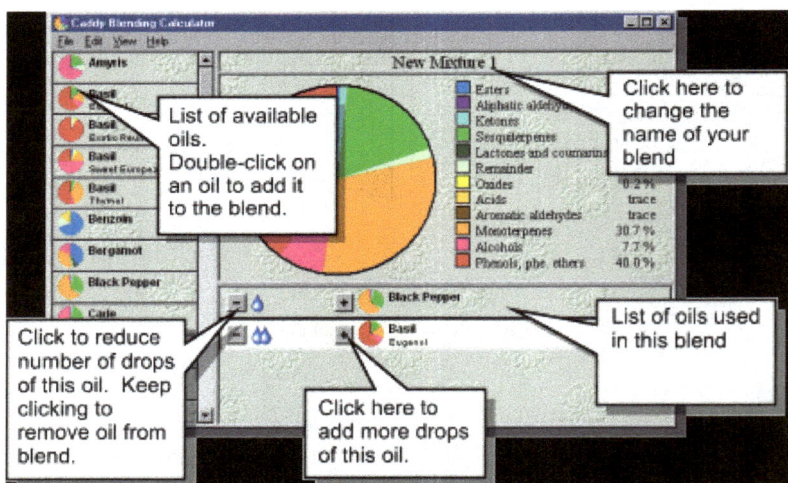

Taken from the book *Essential Oils in Color*:

"Rosemary Caddy graduated from London University with a BSc Honors Degree in Science. As a Reader and Principal Lecturer in Educational Research at Nottingham University, she is the author of a range of educational materials for students of many disciplines. All the materials emphasize visual presentation, enabling students to see, analyze and understand the world around them.

Rosemary is a qualified clinical aromatherapist running her clinic and carrying out a research program on the chemistry of essential oils. She runs lecture courses for aromatherapy students to help them understand and visualize their essential oils. The Caddy Classic Profiles, developed as a result of her research, enable students to enjoy the chemistry of their oils.

Currently, Rosemary is researching the chemistry of synergistic mixes of essential oils."

Aromatherapy and Cancer

There is no evidence that aromatherapy can treat cancer itself. There is some evidence that essential oils may help a person cope with some of the emotional and psychological effects of living with cancer.

Are essential oils carcinogenic?
Phenylpropanoids
- Methyl chavicol/estragole/isoanethole
- Methyl eugenol
- Safrole

A limited number of essential oils have been shown to carry a minimal risk as carcinogenic if swallowed (oral use).

*Topical application is not considered harmful in terms of carcinogenicity.

Pour quality oils or synthetic oils may be a concern.

Do not treat a client for **48** hours after Chemo or Radiation treatment (they are still radioactive and can transfer the toxins to you through skin contact). Aromatherapy benefits people with cancer.

- Anorexia
- Constipation
- Fatigue/weakness
- Nausea
- Odor control
- Peripheral neuropathy
- Respiratory distress
- Stress
- Sweating

Something interesting to think about... When you scrape your elbow, it leaves an area of inflamed skin or a lesion. And a brain lesion is an area of injury or disease within the brain.

My Quantum University "Natural Medicine" course talked about Dr. Ryke Geerd Hamer (17 May 1935 – 2 July 2017), a German doctor practicing in Rome, Italy, and had his license revoked because he claimed he could cure cancer.

By doing a cat scan on his patients, he found that there was always a lesion in the area of the brain that corresponded to where the patient's cancer was in the body. This doctor found that if he focused on curing the cause of the lesion in the brain, it cured the person's cancer.

Bonus:
Hydrotherapy for Pain

Hydrotherapy, aka hydropathy or water cure, is part of an alternative medicine (naturopathy, occupational therapy, and physiotherapy) treatment that uses water for pain relief.

In the 1820s, the Hydropathic Institute of Gafenburg was established and offered a wide variety of water therapies. Sebastian Kneipp (a Bavarian priest and one of the forefathers of the naturopathic medicine movement) managed to treat his health conditions with phytomedicine and fresh water in the 1850s and developed the 'Kneipp Kur', which continues to be studied and practiced today.

Water turns into a solid (ice) at 32° F and vapor (steam) at 212° F. The four factors that contribute to the effects of water on the body are:
- Temperature
- Moisture
- Mineral content
- Mechanical effect (as in the pressure in a shower)

Hydrotherapy can include several techniques, and you can benefit from just one or a combination of them, depending on your symptoms (which may change from session to session); bath, steam shower sessions, sitz baths, foot baths, steam inhalation, hot or cold compresses (or a combination of both being used alternately), body wraps, and cold mitten friction rubs can all be used during a visit to a participating wellness center or spa.

Some of the conditions that can be treated by hydrotherapy include aches and pain, arthritis, depression, headaches and migraines, joint pain, sore and knotted muscles, nerve problems, sleep disorders, acne, cold and flu, stress, and stomach issues.

Essential oils can be used in conjunction with some of hydrotherapy treatments. Peppermint or eucalyptus oil might be added to a steam inhalation session so that the patient can benefit from the heat and the effects of the essential oils.

Rules of Hydrotherapy

Condition	Method	Procedure	Time
Acute 0-72 hours	Cryotherapy (Cold)	13-18°	10-20 minutes
Subacute Early - 2 days Late - 3 weeks	Early - Cool Late - Contrast	Early – 2h:2c, 1x Late - 3h:1c, 3x	12 minutes
Chronic 1 month - years	Thermotherapy (Heat)	42-45°	30 minutes

E.g., Whiplash treatments

- **Acute (first 72 hours) – ice**
- **Subacute (3rd day for 3 weeks) – contrast 3h:1c 3x**
- **Chronic (after swelling is gone) – moist heat**

Aromatherapy has been widely used in water to make steam baths, body wraps, body masks, scrubs, or massages.

- Warmth enhances the absorption of essential oils into the skin.
- Great to add essential oils to the water
  - Compress (wet towel, wring out)
  - Hydrosol
  - Spritzer
  - Massage
  - Baths
  - Body masks or scrubs
  - Body wraps

Always!!! Check if there are any contraindications!!!

Herbal Applications that can benefit hydrotherapy:
- Oatmeal
- Bran
- Salt
- Epsom Salts
- Dead Sea Salts
- Apple cider vinegar
- Sage
- Nutmeg
- Rosemary
- Chamomile
- Pine

- Hayflower
- Oatstraw
- Fennel and nettle
- Ginger
- Sulphur
- Borax, cornstarch, and bicarbonate of soda
- Vitabath & algemarin

CRYOTHERAPY (COLD)

Cryotherapy is any treatment that involves the use of freezing or near-freezing temperatures. Cryotherapy can be delivered to just one area, or you can opt for whole-body cryotherapy.

Localized cryotherapy can be administered in a number of ways, including through ice packs, ice massages, coolant sprays, ice baths, cold towels, and even through probes administered into tissue.

Cold reduces the size of pores and cells, blood vessels to constrict, so bleeding into injured tissues slows, and swelling decreases. Ice causes a reflex action in the muscle spindle, so the damaged muscle relaxes.

Reduces:
- Pain
- arthritic pain,
- inflammation,
- chronic Range of Motion (ROM)
- headaches & migraines
- numbs nerve irritation
- helps treat mood disorders
- atopic dermatitis and other skin conditions
- stops muscle spasm

Risks and Side Effects

The most common side effects of any type of cryotherapy are numbness, tingling, redness, and irritation of the skin. These side effects are almost always temporary *(make an appointment with your doctor if they do not resolve within 24 hours)*.

- Pregnancy
- Heart Conditions
- Very old or very young
- Metal in body
- Cold hypersensitivity
- Cold intolerance
- Cold allergies
- Rheumatoid conditions
- Pectoralis angina
- Raynaud's disease
- Pitted edema
- Diarrhea
- Significant tissue dystrophy
- Previous cold injury (Frostbit)
- Any skin lesions or rashes
- Impaired sensation and paresthesia
- Those with diabetes or any conditions that affect their nerves should not use cryotherapy (the person may be able to feel its effect, which could lead to further nerve damage).

- You should never use cryotherapy for longer than is recommended for the method of therapy you are using.
- For whole-body cryotherapy, no more than four minutes.
- If you are using an ice pack or ice bath at home, you should never apply ice to the area for more than 20 minutes.
- Wrap ice packs in a towel so you do not damage your skin.
- Never performed on a cold or shivering body

CRYOTHERAPY TREATMENTS
Maximum 20 minutes

*All cold therapy begins with the areas furthest from the heart

Cold Pack is used.
- On an acute injury,
- Or after a massage.

Action – lay a cloth down, then place the cold pack, dry naturally

Area – the area of issue

Time – 20 minutes max

Ice Massage is used.
- After deep tissue massage,
- Ligament or tendon inflammation.

Action – freeze water in a small disposable cup (can peel cup as ice melts), massage ice over the area, and dry naturally.

Area – the area of issue

Time – 1 – 30 minutes

Ice on Trigger Points is used.
- During a massage

Action – a piece of plastic wrap is placed over the ice, sweep the ice over the trigger point (do not touch the skin), and dry naturally.

Area – the area of issue

Time – Sweep of cold (10 centimeters per second)

Cold towel/mitt friction is used.
- On an acute injury,
- Or after a massage.

Action - Wet towel friction, repeat, dry rub,

Area – Back, arms, and or legs

Time – Seconds

CONTRAST HYDROTHERAPY

Many people have heard about the Swedish jumping from a hot tub into the snow. This idea is the same with hot and cold water, either dunking a limb or immersing the whole body. The technique is most familiar to serious athletes.

Also known as therapeutic contrasting or vascular flushing, Contrast Hydrotherapy quickly changes tissue temperature from hot to cold and back again and will help with pain and injury rehab (especially repetitive strain injuries).

Contrast constitutes a gentle tissue workout: stimulation without stress and strong sensations without movement.

Effects
- Pain relief
- Muscle relaxation
- Blood flow alterations
- Connective tissue effects
- Body temperature falls

Risks and Side Effects

Contraindicated to apply Contrast Hydrotherapy to an
- Acute injury or an injury that is still swollen, red, hot and/or inflamed.
- Open wounds
- Raynaud's disease
- Pitted edema
- Diarrhea
- Significant tissue dystrophy
- Cancer

CONTRAST TREATMENTS

Action –
- Immersion (sinks, pails, or tubs) is preferred, as the body part is fully surrounded.
- Wrapping (heating pads, thermophores, ice packs, hot and cold towels)
- Spraying or pouring (shower, faucet, or simply pouring from a pail)

Area –

Limbs can be treated most effectively, and because Repetitive Strain Injuries can benefit from Contrast Hydrotherapy, the following conditions are good candidates:
- Carpal Tunnel Syndrome

- Golfers Elbow
- Tennis Elbow
- Plantar Fasciitis
- Achilles Tendonitis
- Shin Splints

Time – Late Subacute 3h:1c, 3x
   Hot for 3 minutes and cold for 1 minute, 3x
- Always end with the cold!
- Cold is always a shorter length of time than hot
Transition as follows:
   - 3 Minutes of comfortably hot
   - 1 Minute of cool, not cold
   - 3 Minutes of hot (hotter than before)
   - 1 Minute of cold (colder than before)
   - 3 Minutes of hot (hotter than before and as hot as you can safely withstand)
   - 1 Minute of cold (colder than before and as cold as you can safely withstand)
   Three alterations between hot and cold are generally recommended.

Footbath
- Flushing effect
- Circulation

Action – have two buckets or bowls, one hot and one cold.

Area – both feet at once

Time –

Transition as follows:
- 3 - 5 Minutes of comfortably hot
- 10 -30 seconds of cool, not cold
- 3 - 5 Minutes of hot
- 10 -30 seconds of cool
- 3 - 5 Minutes of hot
- 10 -30 seconds of cool
- Dry feet

Proceed to a massage or bedrest for 30 minutes

THERMOTHERAPY (HEAT)

No longer than 30 minutes

Today, many people have experienced a sauna or infrared sauna. Dry heat has been proven to allow the body to sweat and release toxins from the skin, stimulate blood circulation, and relax the muscles.

Raising the body's temperature dilates the blood vessels on the surface of the skin, reduces blood pressure, and increases blood flow to the skin and muscles, thus initiating a state of calmness and introspection.

Effects
- Pain relief
- Muscle relaxation
- Blood flow alterations
- Connective tissue effects

Heat is transferred to the tissue in three forms.
- Conduction – hot packs, electric heating pads, paraffin was, hot stones
- Convection – whirlpool and fluidotherapy
- Conversion – ultrasound (physiotherapy)

Risks and Side Effects

Heat is used once the inflammation has gone (usually 72 hours after an injury).

All heat procedures should be protected by using a towel *(sometimes three layers are needed)* between the person and the item of heat.

- Every five minutes, lift the heat, observe the skin under the item, and remove immediately if the area is puffy or mottled or sooner if the client complains.
- Bleeding
- Pregnancy
- Diabetes
- Heart Conditions
- Very old or very young
- Metal in body
- Acute injury
- Inflammation
- Edema or Lymphedema
- Recent or potential hemorrhage
- Fever
- Recent burns, including sunburn
- Any skin lesions or rashes
- Thrombophlebitis
- Impaired sensation and paresthesia
- Hypertension

Temperatures above 113°F (45°C) can cause tissue damage.

*Excellent to heat the area for 10 -15 minutes, then stretch the muscle.

THERMOTHERAPY (HEAT) TREATMENTS

Dry Heat
- Electric pad
  o Under sheets during a massage
- Heated Towels (cover and place on area)
- Heated Gel packs (cover and place on area)
- Microwaved bag (cover and place on area)

Wet or Moist Heat
Before a massage or place where there are chronic aches & pain
- Hot Pack/Hydrocollator Standard Pack (clay pack or silica gel, heated in water) (cover and place on area)
- Water bottle (cover and place on area)
- Hot Rocks (cover and place on area)
- Thai Herbal Compress Balls
- Paraffin wax
- Footbath
- Steam
- Bath
- Towel Compress

Glossary

The information contained in the Glossary is provided for information only.

Abscess – A localized collection of pus in a cavity caused by the breakdown of tissue

Abortifacient – Substance or device used to induce childbirth or premature labor

Acromegaly – Abnormal enlargement of the extremities of the skeleton

Addison's Disease – Hypo functioning of the adrenal cortex

Adrenal Virilism – Excessive output of adrenal hormones

Aerophagia – The abnormal, spasmodic swallowing of air

Alternative – Gradually improves the nutritional state of the body

Amenorrhea – Absence of menses

Anesthetic – Loss of sensation or pain-relieving

Analgesic – Relieves pain

Anaphrodisiac - Diminishing sexual desire

Anaphylaxis – Unusual or exaggerated allergic reaction to a foreign protein or other substances

Andropause – Reduction in male hormones, especially testosterone, resulting in reduced energy, sex drive, and humor. Equivalent of menopause

Anthelmintic – An agent destructive to intestinal worms

Antacid – Combats acid in the body

Antiallergenic – Reduces symptoms of allergy

Antianemic – Counteracting anemia

Antiasthmatic – Countering asthma

Antibacterial – Prevents the multiplication of bacteria

Antibiotic – Combats infection in the body

Anticatarrh – Prevents buildup of mucous in the respiratory tract

Anticoagulant – A substance that prevents the clotting of blood

Anticonvulsive – Controlling convulsions

Antidepressant – Uplifting, counteracting, melancholy

Antidiarrheal – relieves diarrhea

Antidontalgic – Relieving toothache

Antidiuretic – Slows water loss

Antidontalgic – Relieves toothache

Antiemetic – Counteracts nausea, stops or reduces vomiting

Antifungal – Checking the growth of fungi

Antigalactagogic – Impedes flow of milk. Reduces the production of milk secretion in nursing mothers

Antihistamine – A substance that counteracts the effects of histamine. Antihistamines are used to relieve symptoms of allergies

Antilithic – Prevents the formation of stones or calculus

Anti-infectious – Capable of killing infectious agents or stopping spread

Anti-inflammatory – Suppresses inflammation

Antilactogenic – Slows or stops lactation

Antimigraine – Counters migraines

Antimicrobe – Reduces microbes

Antineuralgic – Reduces nerve pain

Antioxidant – A substance that, in small amounts, will inhibit the oxidation of other compounds

Antiparasitic – Acts against parasites

Antipediculotic – Effective against lice

Antiphlogistic – Reduces inflammation

Antiputrefactive – Delays decomposition of animal/vegetable matter

Antiputrescent – Delays decomposition of animal/vegetable matter

Antipruritic – Prevents itching

Antipyretic – Reduces fever

Antipyrotic – Good for the treatment of burns

Antiheumatic – helps relieve rheumatism

Antislcerotic – Prevents hardening of tissue due to chronic inflammation and removes deposits from circulatory vessels

Antiscorbutic – Helps prevent scurvy

Antiseborrheic – Helps prevent excessive discharge from the sebaceous glands

Antiseptic – helps to prevent tissue degeneration and controls infection

Antispasmodic – Relieves cramps

Antisudorific – Reduces sweating

Antitoxin – Produced in the body in response to the presence of a toxin

Antitumoral – Fights tumors

Antitussive – Relieves coughs

Antivenomous – Neutralizes poison

Antiviral – Controls virus organisms

Antizynotic – Stops fermentation

Aperitif – Encouraging appetite

Aphrodisiac – Exciting sexual desire

Aphtha(e) – A small ulcer, such as the small oval or round ulcer covered with a grayish exudate and surrounded by a red halo characteristic

Astringent – Contracts, tightens, and binds tissues

Atelectasis – Collapsed or airless state of the lung, which may be acute or chronic

Bacteriacide – Combating bacteria

Balanitis – Inflammation of the glans penis
Balsamic – healing, soothing, and softening of phlegm

Bechic – Eases coughs

Bright's Disease – see nephritis
Buerger's Disease – Thromboangiitis obliterans. A
disease affecting the medium-sized blood vessels,
particularly the legs' arteries, can cause severe pain. It
can destroy the vessel.

Bronchial Asthma – A condition marked by recurrent
attacks of dyspnea with wheezing due to spasmodic
constriction of the bronchi. This is also known as
Status Asthmaticus, and an acute attack that lasts for
days or weeks can be fatal.

Bronchodilator – Expands a spastic bronchial tube

Calculus – Stones such as renal calculus – kidney
stones

Calmative – Quiet nerves, reduce tension

Candida – Yeast-like fungi commonly part of the
normal flora of the mouth, skin, intestinal tract, and
vagina, but can cause a variety of infections

Carbuncles – An infection of the skin and subcutaneous tissue composed of a cluster of boils

Cardiac – Stimulating effect on the heart

Cardiotonic – Tones the heart muscle

Carminative – Expulsion of gas from the intestines

Catarrh – Inflammation of a mucous membrane with free discharge

Caustic – Burning

Cephalic – Stimulating and clearing the mind

Cervicitis – infection of the cervix

Chilblains – One of the mildest forms of cold injury. It most often occurs on the face, fingers, toes, and ears. Can include swelling, itching, blistering, and ulceration

Cholagogue – Increases flow of bile

Choleretic – Stimulates bile production

Cholecystitis – Inflammation of the gall bladder

Cicatrizant – Helps formation of scar tissue
Coagulant – Clots blood

Colitis – Inflammation of the colon

Conjunctivitis – Inflammation of the conjunctiva or the delicate membrane lining the eyelids and covering the eyeball. Also called "Pink Eye"
Cordial – A tonic to the heart

Cushings Syndrome – A group of serious symptoms that include fatty swellings on the body – moon like fullness in the face, distension of the abdomen, impotence, amenorrhea, high blood pressure, general weakness, unusual growth of hair in females

Cystitis – Inflammation of the urinary bladder

Cytophylactic – Protective of the cells

Decongestant – Releasing nasal mucous

Deodorant – Destroying odour

Demulcent – Soothes irritated tissues, particularly mucous membranes

Depurative – Purifying the blood

Detersive – Detergent. Cleanses wounds and sores and promotes the formation of scar tissue

Detoxicant – Neutralizing toxic substances

Diabetes Insipidus – Insufficient ADH (antidiuretic hormone)

Diabetes Mellitus – A broad term used to denote a complex group of symptoms that have in common a difficulty oxidizing and using glucose, which is secondary to a malfunction of beta cells in the pancreas, whose function is the production of insulin

Diaphoresis – Profuse perspiration

Diaphoretic – causes perspiration

Digestive – Aiding digestion

Disinfectant – Destroying germs

Diuretic – Increasing urine flow

Dysmenorrhoea – Painful menstruation

Dyspepsia – Impairment of the function of digestion

Dyspnea – laboured or difficult breathing

Ecalmpsia – A potentially life-threatening disorder characterized by hypertension, generalized edema, and proteinurea. Convulsive stage of precalmpsia – ecalmpsia syndrome

Ectopic – Gestation development of the ovum in a fallopian tube instead of in the uterus
Emetic – Induces vomiting

Emmenagogic – Promotes and regulates menstrual flow

Emollient – Soothing and softening

Emphysema – A pathologic accumulation of air in tissues or organs. Inspired air is trapped in the lungs, elasticity is lost, and expiration and breathing are difficult

Enuresis – Involuntary discharge of urine

Epithelium (ial) – Cellular covering of internal and external surfaces of the body, including the lining of vessels and other small cavities

Escharotic – used for the treatment of warts

Estrogenic – Similar to estrogen

Eupeptic – Helps release pepsin

Euphoriant – Brings on an exaggerated sense of physical and emotional wellbeing

Exanthematous – Fights rashes

Expectorant – removes excess mucous from the bronchial tubes
Fascia – A sheet or band of fibrous tissue that lies deep to the skin or invests muscles and various organs

Febrifuge – Cooling and reducing high body temperature

Fibrosis – The formation of excessive fibrous tissue

Fixative – Holds a scent or fragrance

Fibrositis – Inflammation of soft tissue, a buildup of urea and lactic acid inside the muscle, causing stiffness and pain

Frigidity – Lacking warmth or feeling

Frochlich's Syndrome – A condition associated with lesions of the hypothalamus and pituitary glands resulting in obesity and sexual infantilism

Fungicide – Destroying fungal infections

Galactagogue – Increasing secretion of milk

Gastralgia – Pain in the stomach

Glossitis – Inflammation of the tongue

Goiter – Enlarged thyroid caused by lack of iodine
Germicide – Kills germs

Gingivitis – A general term for inflammation of the gums. A common symptom is bleeding gums

Grave's Disease – See Hyperthyroidism

Hallucinogen – Induces hallucinations

Hepatic – Stimulates and aids liver and gall bladder function. Related to the liver

Hemophilia – A condition characterized by impaired coagulability of the blood and a strong tendency to bleed

Hemostatic/ Haemostatic – to serve to stop bleeding

Hormonal – Balance or regulates hormone secretions

Hirsutism – Excessive hair on the body and face

Hives – See urticaria

Hydrocele – A painless swelling of the scrotum caused by a collection of fluid in the outermost covering (tunica vaginalis testis) of the testes
Hyperpituitarism – Excessive secretion of hormones. Included Cushing's Syndrome, Acromegaly, and Gigantism

Hyperthyroidism – AKA Grave's Disease – over secretion of the thyroid, resulting in thinness, etc.

Hypertensive – Increasing blood pressure

Hypertropia – Increase in volume of a tissue or organ produced

Hypoglycemia – Lowers blood sugar levels

Hypopituitarism - Deficiency of hormonal production. Includes Dwarfism, Infantilism, and Myxedema

Hypotensive – Lowers blood pressure

Hypothyroidism – Under activity of the gland resulting in fatigue and weight gain

Insecticide – Kills insect pests

Kyphosis – Exaggerated outward curvature of the spine in the thoracic region

Lactogenic – Promotes lactation

Larvicide – Kills insect larvae

Laxative – Aids bowel evacuation

Leucorrhea – Whitish or yellowish viscid (sticky) discharge from the vagina or uterine cavity, which may be a symptom of a disorder either in the reproductive organs or elsewhere in the body. Frequently caused by trichomoniasis (STD)

Leukocytogenic – Encourages the formation of leukocytes

Lipolytic – breaks down fat

Litholytic – Fights the formation of bladder stones

Lordosis – Exaggerated inward curvature in the lumbar region

Mastitis – Inflammation of the breasts, occurring in a variety of forms and degrees of severity

Menorrhagia – Excessive menstruation

Metrorrhea – Abnormal uterine discharge

Musculocutanrous – Pertaining to muscle and skin
Muscular Dystrophy – A painless disease in which the muscles lose protein and fibers. These are replaced by fat and connective tissue. In time, the voluntary muscle system becomes useless

Mucolytic – Destroys or dissolves mucus or an agent that acts so

Myatrophy – Atrophy of a muscle

Myocardial Infarction – Necrosis of the cells of an area of the heart muscle occurring as a result of oxygen deprivation, which in turn is caused by obstruction of the blood supply, aka heart attack

Myosiyis – Inflammation of a muscle

Nervine – reduces nervous disorders and response

Nephritis – An inflammation of the kidney, also called Bright's Disease

Neurasthenia – Neurasthenic neurosis. A neurosis marked by chronic abnormality, fatigability, lack of energy, feelings of inadequacy, moderate depression, inability to concentrate, loss of appetite, and insomnia. Also called nervous prostration.

Neurosis – An emotional disorder that can interfere with a person's ability to lead a normal life

Neurotonic – a tonic for nerves

Ophthalmia – a severe inflammation of the eye

Orchitis – Inflammation of the testis

Ossification – bone hardening

Osteoarthritis – non-inflammatory degenerative joint disease

Osteomalacia – softening of the bones, resulting from impaired mineralization, with excess accumulation of osteoid, caused by vitamin D deficiency in adults. A similar condition in children is called Rickets

Osteoporosis – generalized loss of bone tissue, calcium salts, and collagen in bone

Parasiticide – Kills or repels organisms living on or in a host organism

Paresis – Slight or incomplete paralysis

Parturient – Helps ease delivery in childbirth

Pectoral – Helpful for chest infections

Pediculosis – Treats infestation of lice

Phlebotonic – Tonic to veins

Phlebitis – Inflammation of a vein. In a superficial vein, it is not serious. In a deep vein, it can be more dangerous. Dangerous when it occurs in the cranium

Photosensitizer – An agent that causes heightens sensitivity to sunlight

Pneumothorax – Accumulation of air or gas in the pleural cavity resulting in a collapse of the lung on the affected side

Prophylactic – Helping to prevent disease

Psychoactive – An agent that affects the mind or behavior

Pyelitis – Inflammation of the renal pelvis

Pyorrhea – A copious discharge of pus

Quinsy – Peritonsillar (around the tonsils) abscess
Reiter's Syndrome – Three symptoms comprising urethritis, conjunctivitis, and arthritis, chiefly affecting young men

Resolvent – Dissolves boils and swelling

Restorative – restoring and reviving health

Rheumatoid Arthritis – A chronic systemic disease with inflammatory changes occurring throughout the body's connective tissues

Rickets – A condition of infancy and childhood caused by a deficiency of vitamin D, which leads to altered calcium and phosphorus metabolism and disturbance of the ossification of bone

Rubefacient – An agent that reddens the skin. Increases blood flow.

Scabies – STD commonly called the itch. It is a contagious skin disease caused by the itch mite. Most likely found in the fold of skin as in the groin, under the breasts, and between the fingers and toes.

Scrofula – Formerly the name for TB cervical lymphadenitis

Sedative – Calming
Sialogogue – Inducing the flow of saliva

Spermatitis – Inflammation of the vas deferens

Spermatocele – Cystic distention of the epididymis, containing spermatozoa

Spermatocidal – Destructive to spermatozoa

Spermatocystis – Inflammation of a seminal vessel

Spermatorrhea – Involuntary escape of sperm

Spermolith – A calculus (stone) in the vas deferens

Spermoneuralgia – Neuralgic pain in the spermatic cord

Splenetic – A tonic for the spleen

Splenomegaly – Enlarged spleen

Status Asthmaticus – A condition marked by recurrent attacks of dyspnea with wheezing due to spasmodic constriction of the bronchi. This is known as Bronchial Asthma, and an acute attack can last for days or weeks. It can be fatal.

Stimulant – Increases flow of adrenaline and energy
Stomachic – Relieves gastric disorders

Stupefacient – An agent that induces stupor

Styptic – Arrests external bleeding

Sudorific – Increases perspiration

Syncope – A temporary suspension of consciousness due to cerebral anemia – fainting

Systemic Lupus Erythematosus – A chronic inflammatory disease often febrile and characterized by skin, joints, kidneys, nervous system and mucous membranes injury. It can affect any organ.

Testitis – Inflammation of the testis. Also called orchitis

Thromboangiitis Obliterans – Disease affecting the medium-sized arteries of the leg, which can cause severe pain and, in serious cases, lead to gangrene

Thyroiditis – Inflammation of the thyroid gland

Tonic – Improves bodily performance

Trigeminal Neuralgia – Pain arising from irritation to the fifth
Urethritis – Inflammation of the urethra

Urorrhea – Involuntary flow of urine

Uterotonic – An agent that increases the tone of the uttering muscle

Urticaria – also called hives. Elevated patches of skin that are redder or paler than surrounding skin and they are itchy

Uterine – Tonic to the uterus

Varicocele – Variscocity of the pampiniform Plexus of the spermatic cord, forming scrotal swelling that feels like a bag of worms

Vasodilator – An agent

Vaginitis – Inflammation of the vagina or the sheath

Varicose – Unnaturally and permanently distended veins

Varicosity – A varicose condition

Vasoconstrictor – Contraction of blood vessels

Vasodilator – An agent that causes dilation of blood vessels

Vermifuge – Expulsion of worms

Virucide – An agent that neutralizes a virus

Vulnerary – a plant, drug, etc., for healing wounds

Vulvar Pruritus – Itching of the external genital glands of the female

Bibliography

BIBLIOGRAPHY

Much of this information was created and copywritten when I owned the Canadian Institute of Natural Health And Healing Accredited College. Course information was purchased from Doug and Sue Thomson.

The Fragrant Mind, Valerie Ann Worwood 1996

The Blossoming Heart, Robbi Zeck

The Aromatherapy Bible: The Definitive Guide to Using Essential Oils (Volume 1) by Gill Farrer-Halls

Aromatherapy: Essential Oils in Colour
by Rosemary Caddy | May 1, 1997

Aromatherapy: The Essential Blending Guide
by Rosemary Caddy | Jun 30, 2000

Advanced Aromatherapy: The Science of Essential Oil Therapy by Kurt Schnaubelt, Ph.D. | May 1, 1998

Aromatherapy: Scent and Psyche: Using Essential Oils for Physical and Emotional Well-Being by Peter Damian and Kate Damian | Sep 1, 1995

Ayurveda & Aromatherapy: The EARTH Essentials Guide to Ancient Wisdom and Modern Healing by Light Dr. Miller and Bryan Miller | Feb 14, 1996

The Practice of Aromatherapy: A Classic Compendium of Plant Medicines and Their Healing Properties by Jean Valnet M.D. and Robert B. Tisserand | Jun 1 1982

Aromatherapy for the Soul: Healing the Spirit with Fragrance and Essential Oils by Valerie Ann Worwood | Aug 18, 2006

http://www.bachflower.com/

Gary Young, Young Living Oils

Hydrosols: The Next Aromatherapy by Suzanne Catty | Mar 1, 2001

Massage Therapy Principles and Practice, Susan G. Salvo, 2012

Quantum University, Integrated Medicine - Cancer

BCAOA – British Columbia Alliance of Aromatherapy

References:
Price, Shirley, Price, Len 2002 Aromatherapy for Health Professionals UK: Churchill Livingstone
Schnaubelt, Kurt 1998 Advanced Aromatherapy: The Science of Essential Oil Therapy USA: Healing Arts Press
Read more at Suite101: Essential Oil Quality Testing: Analyzing Aromatherapy Oils for Purity: GC-MS Quality Tests and More
http://aromatherapy.suite101.com/article.cfm/essential_oil_quality_testing#ixzz0pKjtccLT
Essential oils grown in different areas will have a slight difference in the % of a constituent in the essential oil due to chemicals in the earth, heat, wetness, growth period, etc.

Websites:
https://www.aromatics.com/blogs/wellness/chemical-families

http://www.biospiritual-energy-healing.com/hydrotherapy-and-essential-oils.html

https://www.aromaweb.com/articles/parts-of-plants-that-produce-essential-oil.asp

https://theherbalacademy.com/right-lavender-essential-oil/
http://www.newmedicine.ca/

MESSAGE FROM THE AUTHOR

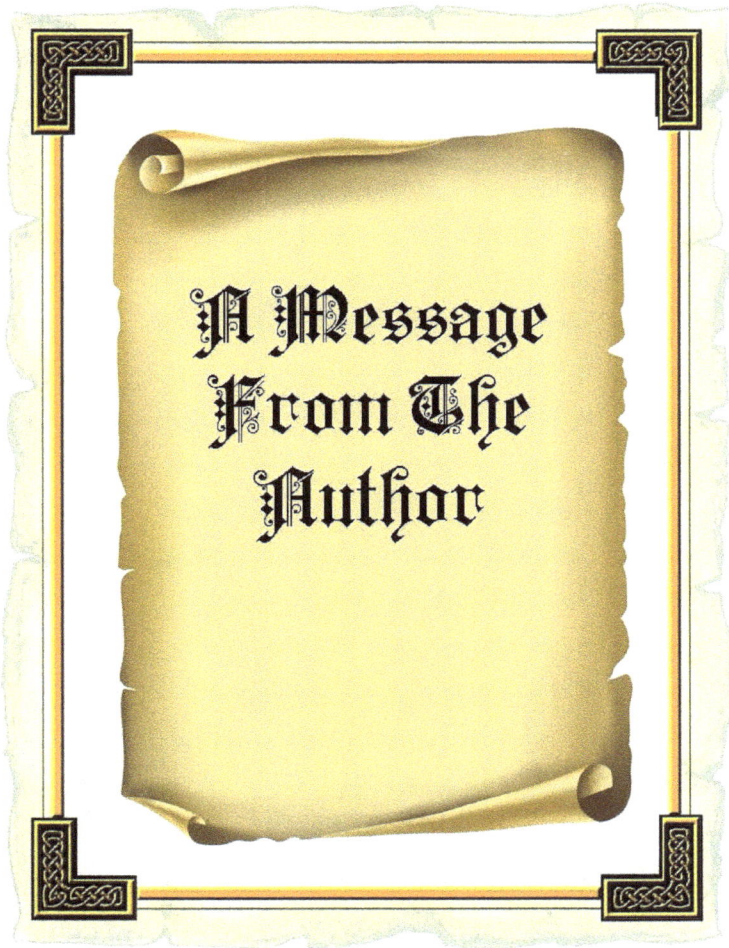

For many years now, Aromatherapy has been one of my favorite modalities. I have used essential oils for soooo many different reasons. It is the next best thing in modern medicine. If I can help myself before I must go to the doctor, I will. Really, it is helping them. That way, they do not have to say, 'If she only looked after herself before this became a problem.'

Constance Santego

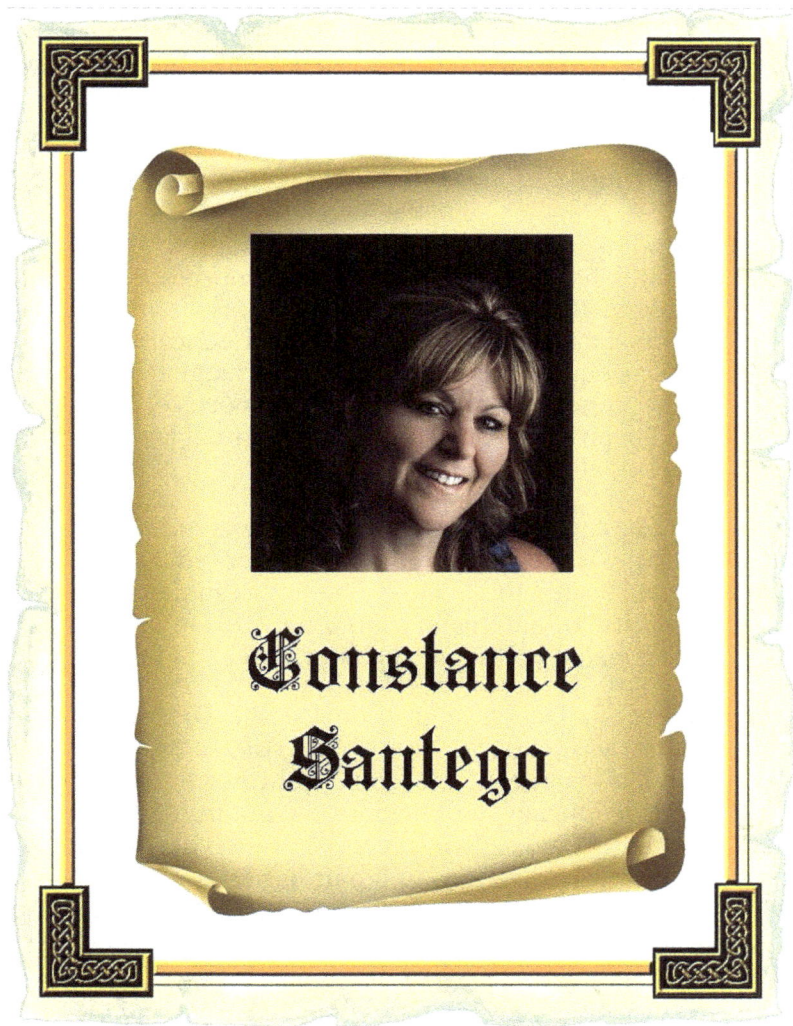

Constance Santego

Dr. Constance Santego is a highly respected expert in the field of holistic health and spiritual healing. With over twenty years of experience teaching courses on these subjects, she has developed a deep understanding of the interconnectedness of the mind, body, and spirit in achieving overall well-being.

Dr. Santego holds a Ph.D. and Doctorate in Natural Medicine, which has provided her with a comprehensive understanding of alternative healing modalities and their application in promoting optimal health. Her educational background has equipped her with the knowledge to address health concerns from a holistic perspective, considering the physical, emotional, and spiritual aspects of an individual's well-being.

Throughout her career, Dr. Santego has been committed to sharing her knowledge and empowering others to take control of their health and healing. She has a unique ability to blend scientific research and traditional wisdom, creating a bridge between conventional and alternative medicine.

In her "Secrets of a Healer" educational series, Dr. Santego draws upon her vast experience and expertise to captivate readers with her insights and teachings. She takes readers on a transformative journey, delving into the realms of holistic health, spirituality, and self-discovery. Through her writing, she aims to inspire individuals to tap into their own innate healing abilities and embrace a balanced and harmonious approach to well-being.

Dr. Santego's work has touched the lives of many, guiding them toward a more profound understanding of themselves and their connection to the world around them. Her series serves as a beacon of wisdom, offering practical tools and techniques for personal growth and transformation.

Overall, Dr. Constance Santego's blend of knowledge, experience, and passion makes her a captivating figure in the field of holistic health and spiritual healing. Her contributions through teaching, writing, and her spellbinding series continue to inspire and empower individuals on their journeys toward well-being and self-discovery.

ALSO AVAILABLE

Play the game Ikona – Discover Your Virtues and Sins

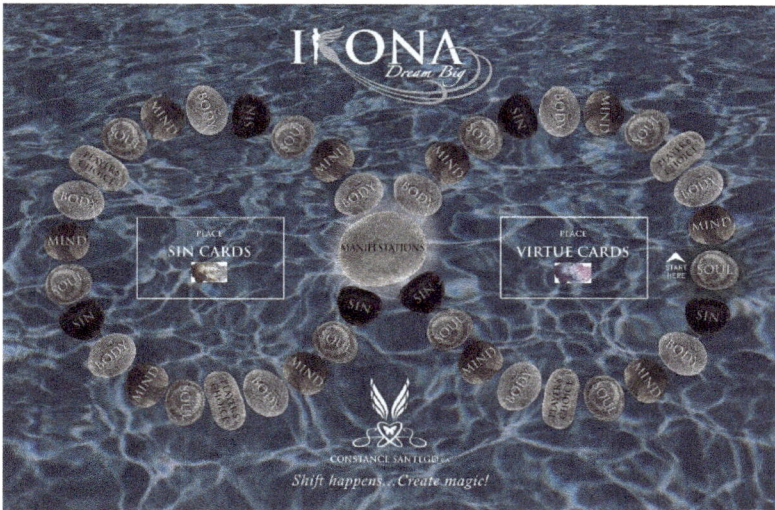

For additional information on

Constance Santego's

wide range of Motivational Products, Coaching Sessions, Spiritual Retreats,
Live Events and Educational Programs

Go to

www.ConstanceSantego.ca

Follow on Instagram - Constance_Santego &
Facebook - constancesantegoo

Subscribe and receive Free Information and Meditations on my
YouTube Channel - Constance Santego

www.ingramcontent.com/pod-product-compliance
Lightning Source LLC
Chambersburg PA
CBHW060316030426
42336CB00011B/1073